Best of Five MCQs for MRCPsych Paper 3

Best of Five MCQs for MRCPsych Paper 3

Lena Palaniyappan
Clinical Lecturer, Division of Psychiatry, University of Nottingham, Nottingham, UK

Rajeev Krishnadas
Clinical Lecturer, Sackler Institute of Psychobiological Research, University of Glasgow, Glasgow, UK

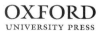
OXFORD
UNIVERSITY PRESS

OXFORD
UNIVERSITY PRESS

Great Clarendon Street, Oxford OX2 6DP

Oxford University Press is a department of the University of Oxford.
It furthers the University's objective of excellence in research, scholarship,
and education by publishing worldwide in

Oxford New York

Auckland Cape Town Dar es Salaam Hong Kong Karachi
Kuala Lumpur Madrid Melbourne Mexico City Nairobi
New Delhi Shanghai Taipei Toronto

With offices in

Argentina Austria Brazil Chile Czech Republic France Greece
Guatemala Hungary Italy Japan Poland Portugal Singapore
South Korea Switzerland Thailand Turkey Ukraine Vietnam

Oxford is a registered trade mark of Oxford University Press
in the UK and in certain other countries

Published in the United States
by Oxford University Press Inc., New York

British Library Cataloguing in Publication Data
Data available

Library of Congress Cataloguing in Publication Data
Data available

Typeset by Glyph International, Bangalore, India
Printed in Great Britain
on acid-free paper by
Ashford Colour Press Limited, Gosport, Hampshire

ISBN 978–0–19–955361–7

10 9 8 7 6 5

FOREWORD

Do you ever look at the breadth of the MRCPsych curriculum and find your heart sinking? As a candidate it can feel that there is just too much to learn – so many topics – so many books and papers – where do you even begin? This book represents an excellent way of starting. It forensically approaches the MRCPsych Paper 3 curriculum and identifies areas that can be easily examined using best of five-style MCQs. Doing this is essential to reduce and focus down on what and how you learn. This book will help you impose a structure on your entire approach to revising for the exam. You can use it both to test what you have learned to date – but also crucially to help you direct and plan your learning also. It will help you focus your reading and learning.

You will learn that that the best approach is to prepare with the exam in mind. This involves both learning the sort of information required and also considering how you will deliver this effectively under exam conditions. Addressing all the component parts of the MCQ and containing 450 questions and answers *Best of Five MCQs for MRCPsych Paper 3* goes a long way towards focusing and structuring your revision. If a candidate used this book to identify key topics and then supplemented the answers here with short additional reading, I believe they would be well-placed to pass this component of the exam.

But of course, knowledge is only one part of passing the exam. The authors know this and provide a helpful overview to the whole exam, and how to prepare for it. Candidates are advised how best to plan their revision, structure their learning, work alone and with others to revise – and reminds readers that there really is life afterwards! It will make it less likely you fail this part of the exam. But if you do, remind yourself why you are interested in psychiatry and in your patients. Step back and try to keep things in perspective, take a holiday, talk to family and friends. Time is a big healer. Then when you're ready, pick the right time to do the exam – that works for you and your life. Sit it for your own reasons rather than because others expect it of you. Use the techniques and focus this book gives you to pass. It will certainly help.

Professor Chris Williams
Professor of Psychosocial Psychiatry
University of Glasgow

ACKNOWLEDGEMENT

This third book in MRCPsych MCQ series has been helped by numerous trainees attending SPMM Course and PassAppraisaL course in London for paper 3 revision. We are grateful for all trainees, who are mostly members of the Royal College of Psychiatrists now, for supporting our work in producing this series.

Special thanks to Dr. Adil Akram for reviewing two chapters (Forensic and General psychiatry) in this book. Dr Rinku Alam provided constructive insight into psychotherapy chapter. Dr Sunanda Ghosh offered very helpful advice on child psychiatry. Dr Rahul Tomar provided immensely practical suggestions in rewriting some questions in the chapter on old age psychiatry. We are grateful to Dr Agnihotri and Dr Chekuri for reviewing the addictions chapter; Dr Jim Crabb and Dr Adam Burnell for reviewing the organic and liaison psychiatry chapter and Dr Everett Julyan for reviewing the psychotherapy. We are indebted to Professor Chris Williams for providing the foreword.

Dr Sree Murthy offered many helpful suggestions throughout the production of this book. Heartfelt thanks to Priya and Sindhu for tolerating our never-ending affairs with the word processors.

CONTENTS

INTRODUCTION

THE MRCPSYCH PAPER 3

MRCPsych exams are the most important exams a psychiatry trainee in the UK will sit during his or her career. Passing the MRCPsych is the most perceptible of the criteria that demonstrate the achievement of a number of competencies during the training. Since spring 2008, there has been a significant change in the pattern of the exam. The structure, syllabus, and the format of questions have changed significantly.

WHO CAN SIT THE EXAM?

The details are clearly given in the Royal College website. They are summarized below for quick reference. Please note that these details are subject to change and so we recommend checking with information at www.rcpsych.ac.uk before you apply.

Training requirements[1,2]
The college has brought out new exam regulations that came into effect on January 2009. Candidates must have completed the mandatory training period of 12 months of post foundation training in psychiatry by the date of sitting the written exams. The recommended time frame for attempting Paper 3 is when the candidate is 18–30 months into training. Posts must be part of a programme of training approved by PMETB OR recognized by the Hospital or Trusts as having specific time, programme (journal clubs, grand rounds, teaching, supervision, etc.), and funds allocated for training. Individual posts can be of either 4 or 6 months' duration. In addition, the college also has placed emphasis on successful completion of annual review of competency progression (ARCP) and other workplace based assessments (WPBA) to be eligible for training. The exact details need be confirmed from the college website as they are subject to regular reviews.

WHAT IS PAPER 3?

The MRCPsych Paper 3 is 3 hours long and contains 200 questions. The paper consists of multiple choice questions (MCQs = 75%) and extended matching items (EMI = 25%). MCQs are in the 'best of five' (BOF) format. A BOF MCQ comprises a question stem of varying length, followed by a list of five options. Candidates should choose the single best option that answers the question.

The college has retained the EMI format from the previous pattern in the new format. An EMI comprises of a specific theme (sometimes with a short description), followed by a set of answer choices (often in an alphabetical order) and a lead-in statement explaining what the candidate is being asked to do. This lead-in statement is then followed by a question list, set out in a logical order. The questions may be asked in form of clinical vignettes. The candidate may be required to choose more than one answer from the list of options for an individual question; in this case, the number of correct options will be clearly marked adjacent to the question.

Breakdown of questions, Paper 3 (Clinical Topics)
The Clinical Topics will be approximately two-thirds of the paper. The Critical Review component will make up approximately one-third of the paper.

General adult psychiatry   32%
- Classification of disease, preventative strategies
- Presentation of illness and treatment
- Hospital liaison psychiatry
- Neuropsychiatry
- Medicine relevant to psychiatry and HIV
- Research

Old age psychiatry   15%
Addictions   11%
Child and adolescent psychiatry   15%
Forensic psychiatry   9%
Learning disability   10%
Psychotherapy and psychopathology   8%

HOW TO PREPARE FOR THE EXAM

The MRCPsych journey starts the very day the training starts. Preparation should be directed towards gaining the requirements towards sitting the exam, as well as getting a good knowledge of the theories that underlie the principles and practice of psychiatry. Preparation for the exams should be cumulative – i.e. the knowledge gained during the preparation for papers 1 and 2 should ideally contribute to your performance in paper 3. The college makes it clear that that the emphasis for paper 3 is going to be on clinical topics. So it is likely that a person, who has had a mixture of experience in specialty posts, such as forensics, addictions, psychotherapy, and learning disability, would be at advantage. Those who have not had the opportunity to spend time in specialty areas may find it difficult to get time to read these topics. It is essential that these topics don't get left out.

A topic that may get left out, because it is not specifically attended to is critical appraisal. Critical appraisal of research is a core skill that is to be developed early on in training. This is essential to understand the rationale behind our daily 'evidence-based practice'. This could be best done by arranging focused 'journal clubs' with special emphasis on critical appraisal with a specific type of research article on each occasion. For example, if there are six trainees in a unit, they could divide topics among themselves, so that each person gets the opportunity to prepare and present a particular type of research paper each week. So if the first trainee presents a paper on a randomized controlled trial, the second person presents a paper on meta-analysis the following week, the third person presents a paper on economic analysis in the third week, etc. This would also mean that each person would be an expert in the type of paper he/she presented and can impart the knowledge to others. Focused journal clubs can be particularly difficult to organize and will need full cooperation from the consultants, college tutor and most of all, the trainees in the unit. This can be very difficult to organize as often journal clubs lack orientation and structure. This is complicated by the fact that the more junior trainees and General Practice trainees may not be interested in an exam-focused critical appraisal at all. If it is difficult to arrange at a hospital site level, it would be best to arrange this among the candidates themselves during group study time.

Eight to 10 weeks towards the exam, the candidate is expected to have read a core textbook in psychiatry – cover to cover – for example the *Oxford Shorter Textbook of Psychiatry* or the *Companion to Psychiatric Studies*. During the final 8–10 weeks preceding the exam, it would be best to create a timetable with the syllabus and curriculum in mind so as not to leave out important topics. Reading during this period should be exam oriented and should be done along with practice MCQs. This could be done on your own or in a study group. Preparing in a group helps to get an idea of where one stands with respect to the knowledge base.

Practice tests

A number of revision courses are now available for the new MRCPsych exams. Revision courses and materials should be used only to aid rapid revision and synthesize exam techniques. It is best to revise from material the candidate has already read once through the previous 10 months, rather than starting afresh. The MRCPsych exam prepares a psychiatric trainee for lifelong learning. It is best not to rely exclusively on 1 or 2 days of cramming to gain knowledge that sets your career on track.

It is best to take a number of mock and practice tests before the exam, as these will give a fairly good idea of strengths and weaknesses. Look out for mock exams conducted by industry sponsors and local tutors. If possible, request your senior colleagues to organize a mock exam. It is best to do mock exams in the original exam conditions, i.e. in paper and pencil format, with 200 questions and a time of 180 minutes.

Books to read

Knowledge is not derived from textbooks alone. All kinds of resources are useful, including the internet, but it is best to base the core reading on standard textbooks. These textbooks should form the basis of reading, but reading should not be restricted to these.

The two reference books that we recommend are *Kaplan and Sadock's Comprehensive Textbook of Psychiatry* (this is an American book, which is comprehensive, with DSM and ICD criteria, and forms excellent reading in all aspects of psychiatry, including specialty topics) and the *New Oxford Textbook of Psychiatry* (the latest edition is now published). Both are two-volume textbooks and are useful for all parts of the exams.

For 'core' text reading, the *Shorter Oxford Textbook of Psychiatry* is a very good book. Each chapter is written in an authoritative style and relevant to training in the UK. At the end of each section or topic there is a reference for further reading in the topic, which is invaluable. Most psychiatric specialty topics are covered extensively in the above-mentioned textbooks. A relatively new book that has been published recently and highly recommended by the authors is the *Essential Psychiatry* textbook edited by Robin Murray, *et al.* This book is very much UK oriented, but with a fantastic array of authors from both sides of the pond, the book gives a concise and truly international view of psychiatry. A special recommendation by the authors is *Sadock's Synopsis of Psychiatry*. This remains one of the most comprehensive 'short' textbooks of psychiatry. Any one of these 'core' books should ideally be read, cover to cover, at least once over the period of training.

The Oxford specialist handbooks in psychiatry are currently available for child psychiatry, addictions, and old age psychiatry. The books are a concise overview of the relevant clinical topics. The *seminar* series brought out by the college are authoritative in each specialty. Since these books are brought out by the Royal College, it seems logical to think that a number of questions may be based on these books. It should be kept in mind that some of these books are outdated.

The *Handbook of Liaison Psychiatry* edited by Lloyd and Guthrie is recommended as a reference text for liaison psychiatry. *Lishman's Organic Psychiatry* has been recently updated and forms a good reference source for neuropsychiatry. The authors recommend *Neuropsychiatry and Behavioural Neuroscience* by Jeffrey Cummings as a concise and to the point book for neuropsychiatry. The *Oxford textbook of Old age Psychiatry* edited by Jacoby, *et al.* is a standard reference textbook for old age psychiatry.

As far as child psychiatry is concerned, *Goodman and Scott's – Child Psychiatry* is the standard recommended read at the basic training level. Sir Michael Rutter's textbook *Child and Adolescent Psychiatry* remains a classic reference textbook. We also recommend Lewis's *Child and Adolescent Psychiatry: A Comprehensive Textbook* edited by Martin and Volkmar. It is an American book, but is an excellent and comprehensive read. Topics on substance use are very well covered in Kaplan and Sadock's *Synopsis of Psychiatry*. There is a separate chapter dedicated for each substance and psychopathology associated with their use.

Most core psychotherapy topics can be read from any standard textbook of general psychiatry. Both the two-volume reference books mentioned earlier have extensive chapters on psychotherapy. Two other books are the *Oxford textbook of Psychotherapy* and *Gabbard's Textbook of Psychotherapeutic Treatments*. The college *seminar* series is concise and Freeman and Power's *Handbook of Evidence-based Psychotherapies* gives a good critical appraisal of most psychotherapeutic research.

The Royal College's own *Advances in Psychiatric Treatment* is a good source for review articles, in most cases written by experts in the field. Nevertheless, it should be noted these are mostly narrative rather than systematic reviews.

The *Evidence-based Mental Health Journal* is an excellent source for articles on critical appraisal. The *Canadian Journal of Psychiatry* (not very popular in Britain, but available free of charge online) is an excellent source for up-to-date review articles and also for articles on critical appraisal and statistical concepts. The author of the statistics topics in the journal – David Streiner – is an excellent writer, who makes these often complex topics highly accessible to we clinicians, most of us suffering from 'photonumerophobia' (a fear that our fear of numbers would come to light – a concept devised by Streiner).

MRCPsych exam Paper 3 revision techniques in summary

1. Always stick to the standard textbooks you have read earlier. But remember textbooks are not written with the aim of helping trainees pass MRCPsych exams. So avoid spending too much time on irrelevant details. Nevertheless, you should have read a 'core' textbook, cover to cover, at least 8 weeks before the exam.
2. As the question banks evolve, the candidate should be able to revise and attempt the exam confidently; one should get the basic concepts straight and correct, in order to tackle any surprises!
3. Group study helps in many ways; but make sure your peers are motivated to fully participate in the groups (especially for critical appraisal discussions).
4. Plan, plan, and plan! Structure your time according to the syllabus you have to revise. Spend equal time updating your knowledge from journals and solving MCQs.
5. There is no harm in utilizing all available materials before you attempt your exam – ask your senior ST trainees or colleagues and seek resources from revision courses and local MRCPsych teaching lectures.
6. A word of caution, most senior psychiatrists have a vast amount of clinical wisdom. Clinical wisdom is gained over a period of time, having spent a number of years working in the specialty and may be extremely helpful in the day-to-day practice of psychiatry. While this can be useful in topics like psychotherapy and the likes, it is best to stick to standard reference textbooks as sources of information for a theory exam like the MRCPsych, which bases a lot of its questions on recent advances and evidence-based sources.

APPROACH TO MULTIPLE CHOICE QUESTIONS[3,4]

The MRCPsych exam is more than reading and understanding the core subject, it is also to do with the technique of attempting the best of five MCQs. Unlike the old-style ISQ, the new style is a bit more difficult to do because the chance of getting the answer wrong is 80% compared to 50% with the older style. The very concept of selecting the best answer lies in the fact that there may be more than one right answer, but we need to choose the best answer. In order to do this you get 180 minutes to answer 200 questions, that is less than 1 minute to answer a question. This means that the more familiar you are with the concepts, the faster you can answer and you will be able to spend more time on the more difficult and longer questions. It is said that in most medical examinations, candidates who answer half the questions correctly would score around the 50th or 60th percentile. A score of 65% (130/200) would place the examinee above the 80th percentile, whereas a score of 30% (60/200) would rank him or her below the 15th percentile. Test performance will always be

influenced by your test-taking skills. Considering various test-taking strategies, developing and perfecting them well in advance of the test date can help you concentrate better on the test itself. We recommend you try various techniques to find what works best for you. It should, in the end, help you to:
- increase your reading pace;
- focus on the most relevant information;
- eliminate as many options when you are not sure of the correct answer.

You require enough practice using the techniques so that it becomes second nature and you don't concentrate on anything but how to choose the correct answer when you actually sit the exam.

Timing

Time management is an important skill for exam success. As mentioned above, the test has 200 questions to be answered in 3 hours. This leaves less than a minute for each question. Each time you spend more than a minute on a single question, time should be made up on other questions. Therefore it is essential to practise answering questions within a time limit to avoid pacing errors in the exam. This is where attempting a number of mock exams will help.

Approaching each question

There are several established techniques for tackling MCQs which will help you in finding the single best answer choice. One of these is classifying each question as easy, workable, or impossible. The basic aim in doing this is to
- answer all easy questions;
- figure out the answer to all the workable questions in a reasonable amount of time;
- make fast and intelligent guesses on the impossible ones.

Another technique is to read the answer choices first along with the last sentence of the question before reading through the question quickly, so as to extract the most relevant information as well as to consider each of the answer possibilities in the context of the question. This is especially relevant when the question stem is large, for example a case scenario.

Elimination is one of the best tools that can be used in a single best answer multiple choice exam.

Excluding the possibility of one answer choice proportionately increases the probability of you choosing the right answer.

Since this is a paper and pencil exam, it is better to answer the questions in order, one by one; this reduces chances of skipping and accidentally marking the wrong question or skipping an item. To avoid these 'frame-shift' errors, answer difficult questions with your best guess, mark them for review, move on and come back to them if you have time at the end.

Random guessing

- There are no negative marks for wrong answers, so no question should be left unanswered.
- A hunch is probably better than a random guess; we also suggest selecting a choice which you recognise over another which is totally unfamiliar to you.
- It is never beneficial to pick random choices unless you are grossly out of time and not answering all the questions, in which case the best bet would be to select a single letter like 'C' and marking the remaining questions with it. It is obvious that in this case the chance of picking the correct answer decreases with more answer choices. It is also believed that MCQ makers prefer to hide the answers either in C or D, the middle-most choices, more often than in the periphery (however, it should be noted that the college is trying to get rid of this bias by presenting the multiple choices in alphabetical order).
- It is also very important to not randomly guess the answers during your study and review sessions as well as the practice test sessions, as it may increase the tendency to do the same for the exam.

- As mentioned before, it is essential to take as many practice tests as possible to try the various techniques and select the ones that give you the best results.
- Use any extra time you might have to recheck your answers. Do not be casual in your review or you may overlook serious mistakes.
- Never give up. If you begin to feel frustrated try taking a 30-second breather. Remember your goals and keep in mind the effort and time you have spent in preparing for the exam compared with the small additional effort you will need to keep your focus and concentration throughout the exam.

Other things to do before the exam

Make arrangements for study leaves as early as possible. It is also important to find out how much private study leave you are entitled to. Make all the necessary swaps on the on call rota. Some deaneries arrange for stay and transport for the exam if there are a number of candidates taking the exam. Application forms should be sent well in time. If there are queries regarding applications, they should be clarified from the college at the earliest.

The day prior to exam, choose a good place to stay near the centre, even if it is expensive. As usual, it is important to get a good night's sleep. A good preparation should make you feel confident.

BOF MCQ exam techniques in summary

1. People who fail in MCQ exams do so not because they don't know the answer for some questions; it is because they think they know the answer and keep thinking about one question for 5 minutes or so, losing the remaining time to answer the rest.
2. All questions carry one mark only, no matter how easy or difficult each one is. So why spend all your time on 'difficult ones'?
3. In large, clinical vignette type of questions you may have many irrelevant details; at the same time you may also have valuable clues to solve the BOF. It is useful to read the last sentence of the question, quickly before reading the large vignettes fully.
4. People have different styles of approaching BOF. Exclusion technique needs more time than direct answer picking; if your style is one of exclusion, make sure you practise well enough to carry this out faster during the exam.

AFTER THE EXAM

If you have some stamina left at the end of this huge ordeal, it is not a bad idea to start recollecting the questions to form a question bank which will be useful for future candidates. It is best to recollect the questions in the company of a couple of colleagues. It will be a good idea to get the questions back to the college tutor and this will help to arrange further teaching. This will also help you to prepare for paper 3 in future.

READING LIST

Reference books and core clinical psychiatry:
Gelder MG, *et al.*, eds. *Shorter Oxford Textbook of Psychiatry*, 5th edn. Oxford University Press, 2006.
Sadock BJ and Sadock VA. *Kaplan and Sadock's Synopsis of Psychiatry: Behavioral Sciences/Clinical Psychiatry*, 10th edn. Lippincott Williams and Wilkins, 2007.
Murray RM, Kendler KS, McGuffin P, *et al.*, (2008). *Essential Psychiatry*, 4th edn. Cambridge University Press.
Gelder MG, *et al.*, eds. *New Oxford Textbook of Psychiatry*. Oxford University Press, 2009.
Sadock BJ and Sadock VA, eds. *Kaplan and Sadock's Comprehensive Textbook of Psychiatry* (2 Vol. set) 9th edn. Lippincott Williams and Wilkins, 2009.

Neuropsychiatry and Liaison psychiatry
Lloyd G and Guthrie E. Handbook of Liaison Psychiatry, 1st edn. Cambridge University Press, 2007.
Cummings JL and Mega MS, eds. *Neuropsychiatry and Behavioural Neuroscience*. Oxford University Press, 2003.

Research methodology and critical appraisal
Lawrie S, McIntosh A, and Rao S. *Critical Appraisal for Psychiatrists* (MRCPsy Study Guides) (Paperback 2000). This is a good book, slightly more detailed, with MCQs for exercise.
Norman GR and Streiner DL. *Biostatistics: the Bare Essentials*, 3rd edn. BC Decker, 2007. This is good book on statistics, written for doctors with knowledge of mathematics at no greater than high school level.
Greenhalgh T. *How to Read a Paper: The Basics of Evidence-based Medicine*, 3rd edn. Blackwell, 2006.
Evidence-Based Mental Health Journal (available through Athens accounts) and Review articles in the *Canadian Journal of Psychiatry* are highly recommended.
www.passappraisal.com is a good resource maintained by the authors.

Child and adolescent psychiatry
Rutter SM, Bishop D, Pine D, *et al. Rutter's Child and Adolescent Psychiatry*, 5th edn. WileyBlackwell, 2008.
Volkmar AMFR. *Lewis's Child and Adolescent Psychiatry: A Comprehensive Textbook*, 4th edn. Lippincott Williams & Wilkins, 2007.
Goodman R and Scott S. *Child Psychiatry*, 2nd edn. WileyBlackwell, 2005.

Old age psychiatry
Jacoby R, Oppenheimer C, Dening T, and Thomas A. *Oxford Textbook of Old Age Psychiatry*, 4th edn. Oxford University Press, 2008.
Sheehan B, Karim S, and Burns A. Old Age Psychiatry, 1st edn. Oxford University Press 2009.

Psychotherapy
Gabbard GO, Beck JS, and Holmes J. *Oxford Textbook of Psychotherapy*. Oxford University Press, 2007.
Gabbard GO. *Textbook of Psychotherapeutic Treatments in Psychiatry*, 1st edn. American Psychiatric Publishing, 2008.
Naismith J and Grant S. *Seminars in the Psychotherapies*. Gaskell, 2007.
Freeman C and Power M. *Handbook of Evidence-based Psychotherapies: A Guide for Research and Practice*, 1st edn. WileyBlackwell, 2007.

[1] http://rcpsych.ac.uk/PDF/Exams%20Eligibility%20July%202008.pdf
[2] http://rcpsych.ac.uk/exams/about/mrcpsychpaperiii.aspx
[3] Bhushan V, Le T. First Aid for the USMLE Step 1 (First Aid) (Paperback) McGraw Hill Higher Education; 16Rev Ed edition (1 Jan 2006)
[4] Princeton Review, Stein M, Hwang G. Cracking the Boards: USMLE Step 1, 3rd Edition (Princeton Review Series) (Paperback) Princeton Review; 3 edition (Dec 2000)

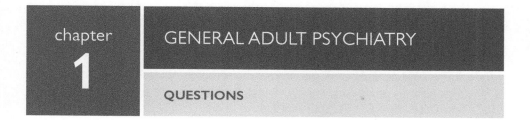

1. **According to ICD-10 criteria which of the following is considered to be the minimum required weight loss to be significant as a diagnostic criteria for somatic syndrome associated with depression?**

   A. Loss of 1% body weight in 1 month
   B. Loss of 5% body weight in 3 months
   C. Loss of 2% body weight in 2 weeks
   D. Loss of 5% body weight in 1 month
   E. Loss of 15% body weight in 1 week

2. **The prevalence of catatonic phenomenon among patients with schizophrenia is estimated to be around**

   A. 1–2%
   B. 0.01–0.05%
   C. 5–10%
   D. 15–25%
   E. 30–35%

3. **Seasonal affective disorder (SAD) is a popular concept but not formally considered as a separate category under current classificatory systems. Which of the following statements is true with regard to this condition?**

   A. Seasonal depression carries higher familial risk of affective disorders than non-seasonal depression
   B. In phototherapy for SAD, exposure to skin is more effective than exposure to eye
   C. Early-morning light therapy is more effective than evening exposure
   D. Side-effects of exposure are more intense with evening than morning therapy
   E. Conventional antidepressants have no effect on seasonal depression

4. **The 1-year prevalence of dysthymia is estimated to be around**

   A. 15–20%
   B. 20–25%
   C. 1–6%
   D. 0.1–0.6%
   E. 10–15%

5. **The most powerful predictors of recurrence of depressive episodes among the following is**
    A. Previous episodes of depression and presence of residual symptoms
    B. Non-bipolar diagnosis and later age of onset
    C. Female gender and earlier age of onset
    D. Higher degree of life events and family history of affective disorders
    E. Male gender and past history of psychiatric admission

6. **The proportion of patients who develop a depressive episode and then go on to develop an episode of mania within 10 years is approximately**
    A. 1 in 2
    B. 1 in 10
    C. 1 in 4
    D. 1 in 50
    E. 1 in 200

7. **Clinical depression and bereavement share many common features. Which of the following clinical features points to clinical depression rather than normal mourning?**
    A. Brief hallucinations
    B. Somatic symptoms
    C. Anxiety when reminded of loss
    D. Psychomotor retardation
    E. Angry pining

8. **Which of the following is an early sign of prolonged grief?**
    A. Self-blame regarding the death
    B. Shock and disbelief
    C. Clinging behaviour
    D. Anxiety when reminded of loss
    E. Brief hallucinations

9. **The term 'specifier' is used when describing psychiatric diagnoses. Which of the following is correct with regard to this term?**
    A. It is used in ICD-10 only
    B. It is used in DSM-IV only
    C. It refers to treatment response
    D. It is used in both DSM IV and ICD 10
    E. It refers to number of previous episodes

10. **Which of the following is true with regard to the longitudinal course of bipolar disorder?**
    A. The duration of mood episodes decreases progressively
    B. Initial episodes have more rapid onset than later episodes
    C. The interval between episodes decreases progressively
    D. Seasonal pattern is more common in bipolar type 1 than type 2
    E. Later episodes are more likely to be triggered by life events than the initial episodes

11. **The most common psychiatric disturbance associated with Cushing's disease is**
    A. Depression
    B. Mania
    C. Mixed affective state
    D. Schizophreniform psychosis
    E. Dementia

12. **Polyuria can be a troublesome side-effect with lithium therapy. Which of the following is NOT correct with response to lithium-related polyuria?**
    A. It is seen in one-third of those treated with lithium
    B. It is usually reversible
    C. Once-daily dose produces more polyuria than multiple doses a day
    D. Amiloride is a useful intervention
    E. Dose reduction may alleviate polyuria

13. **Which of the following electrolyte disturbances simulate lithium-induced changes in electrocardiogram?**
    A. Hyperkalaemia
    B. Hypocalcaemia
    C. Hypomagnesaemia
    D. Hypokalaemia
    E. Hyponatraemia

14. **Lithium is associated with thyroid dysfunction in some cases. Which of the following is false with respect to this association?**
    A. 5–10% of patients on lithium develop clinical hypothyroidism
    B. Thyroid enlargement is the most common clinical presentation
    C. Presence of thyroid antibodies increases the risk
    D. Family history of thyroid disease increases the risk
    E. Increased TSH is the most sensitive laboratory index

15. **Compared with the general population, the risk of Ebstein's anomaly in children of mothers exposed to lithium during the first trimester of pregnancy is**
    A. 2–3 times higher
    B. 10–20 times higher
    C. 50–80 times higher
    D. 100–120 times higher
    E. 4–5 times higher

16. **A 48-year-old man is prescribed sodium valproate for prophylaxis against bipolar mania. He develops a confusional state despite liver function tests being within the normal range. Which of the following conditions related to valproate use is most likely to be associated with the above presentation?**
    A. Hyperammonaemia
    B. Hepatic failure
    C. Pancreatitis
    D. Hypertensive encephalopathy
    E. Ketoacidosis

17. **All of the following patients are under carbamazepine therapy for bipolar disorder. In which of the following patients will you discontinue the carbamazepine treatment immediately?**
    A. A 34-year-old man developing dizziness
    B. A 50-year-old man with blood carbamazepine levels 9 mg/L
    C. A 44-year-old woman with neutrophil count less than 1000 per mm^3
    D. A 37-year-old man with sodium levels 129 mEq/dL
    E A 48-year-old woman with elevation of thyroid-stimulating hormone (TSH) levels

18. **Which of the following predicts a good prophylactic effect of lithium in bipolar disorder?**
    A. Absence of family history of bipolar disorder
    B. Presence of neurological signs
    C. 'Depression–mania–well interval' pattern of bipolar course
    D. Good antimanic efficacy during acute episode
    E. Absence of complete inter-episode recovery

19. **Which of the following situations associated with parental loss carries the highest risk of developing depression as an adult?**
    A. Children born to single mothers
    B. Children of divorced mothers
    C. Children of remarried mothers with conflicts after remarriage
    D. Childhood bereavement with loss of one parent
    E. Children living with divorced parent after conflictual relationship

20. **Adverse life events are consistently associated with depression. Which of the following statements with respect to the above relationship is NOT true?**
    A. 30% of those with depression have no history of preceding significant life events
    B. Suicide attempters have a higher amount of life events than depressed patients
    C. Loss or humiliation events are highly correlated with depression
    D. The impact of life events depends on the contextual threat posed by them
    E. No reverse causality exists between depression and life events

21. **All of the following are characteristic features of a depression-prone individual except**
    A. Perceiving higher probability for aversive outcomes
    B. Believing that aversive events are uncontrollable
    C. Attributing negative events to external, unstable but specific causes
    D. Fragile self-esteem
    E. Harbouring high amount of information processing biases

22. **Anti-obesity drug rimonabant is associated with significant psychiatric adverse effects. Which of the following correctly describes the mechanism of action of rimonabant?**
    A. Cannabinoid CB_1-receptor antagonist
    B. Cannabinoid CB_2-receptor antagonist
    C. Monoclonal antibody against $GABA_A$ subunits
    D. NMDA receptor antagonist
    E. Cholecystokinin antagonist

23. **Which of the following neurotransmitters is proposed to be involved in increasing the significance (salience) of external stimuli in patients with schizophrenia?**
    A. GABA
    B. Glutamate
    C. Endocannabinoids
    D. Dopamine
    E. Noradrenaline

24. **All of the following are diagnostic features of neuroleptic malignant syndrome (NMS) except**
    A. Diaphoresis
    B. Fluctuant blood pressure
    C. Myoclonus
    D. Tachycardia
    E. Mutism

25. **The most common phase of sleep when nocturnal panic attacks appear is**
    A. Transition between stage 2 and stage 3
    B. Transition between stage 1 and stage 2
    C. REM sleep
    D. Transition between REM sleep and awake state
    E. Stage 1 sleep

26. **All of the following are sleep changes associated with depression except**
    A. Reduced REM latency
    B. Reduced REM density
    C. Increased duration of first REM period
    D. Low arousal threshold
    E. Reduced stage 3 and 4 sleep

27. **A 60-year-old man has episodes of disturbed sleep. He experiences unusual movements associated with singing and talking to unseen people during some of these episodes. He recalls vivid dreams when he wakes up. The most appropriate diagnosis would be**
    A. Sleep-walking
    B. Sleep terrors
    C. REM sleep behavioural disorder
    D. Periodic limb movement disorder
    E. Restless legs syndrome

28. **All of the following are recognized treatment options for restless legs syndrome except**
    A. Levodopa
    B. Pergolide
    C. Pramipexole
    D. Amitriptyline
    E. Clonazepam

29. **A 29-year-old man presents with erectile dysfunction. His history reveals excessive stress at work. Which of the following indicates a psychogenic rather than an organic cause for his sexual dysfunction?**
    A. Sudden onset of the erectile problem
    B. Erectile dysfunction occurs in all settings
    C. Loss of early-morning erections
    D. Preserved ejaculation despite impaired erection
    E. Complete lack of tumescence

30. **Which of the following drugs used for erectile dysfunction acts via the dopaminergic mechanism?**

    A. Sildenafil
    B. Vardenafil
    C. Alprostadil
    D. Apomorphine
    E. Yohimbine

31. **Which of the following instruments is validated for predictive screening for chronic post-traumatic stress disorder (PTSD) in those who are exposed to traumatic events?**

    A. Holmes and Rahe Social Adjustment scale
    B. Life Events and Difficulties Scale
    C. Trauma Screening Questionnaire
    D. Appraisal of Life Events Scale
    E. Abbreviated Injury Scale

32. **Reduced flush response to nicotinic acid (niacin) skin patches has been demonstrated in**

    A. Depression
    B. Bipolar disorder
    C. Schizophrenia
    D. Autism
    E. Anorexia nervosa

33. **Oral administration of a tryptophan-free amino acid mixture can lead to tryptophan depletion. This can trigger relapse of depression in patients being treated for depression. The above phenomenon is most likely seen in those on**

    A. Selective serotonin reuptake inhibitors (SSRIs)
    B. Tricyclic antidepressants
    C. Reboxetine
    D. Cognitive behavioural therapy
    E. Maintenance electroconvulsive therapy

34. **All of the following receptor changes are correctly paired except**

    A. Increased cortical $5HT_{2A}$: depressed patients
    B. Increased cortical $5HT_{1A}$: depressed patients
    C. Increased cortical $5HT_{2A}$: ECT treatment
    D. Increased cortical $5HT_{2A}$: suicide victims
    E. Decreased β receptors: antidepressant therapy

35. **Which of the following is true with regard to lithium toxicity?**

    A. Severity is highly correlated with serum levels

    B. Neurotoxicity occurs only above therapeutic serum levels

    C. Fine tremor is a sign of toxicity

    D. Lithium levels often rise even after cessation of treatment

    E. Most patients are left with some residual neurological damage

36. **Which of the following antidepressants demonstrate the highest affinity for muscarinic acetylcholine receptors of the human brain?**

    A. Amitriptyline

    B. Clomipramine

    C. Amoxapine

    D. Trazodone

    E. Desipramine

37. **The number of patients who die from hypertensive crises (including fatal 'cheese reaction') when monoamine oxidase inhibitors such as tranylcypromine are prescribed is approximately**

    A. 1 in 1000 patients

    B. 1 in 100 patients

    C. 1 in 10 000 patients

    D. 1 in 100 000 patients

    E. 1 in 10 patients

38. **Which of the following antidepressants has been found to be as lethal as tricyclic antidepressants (TCAs) in cases of overdose?**

    A. Citalopram

    B. Mirtazapine

    C. Venlafaxine

    D. Moclobemide

    E. Escitalopram

39. **The lorazepam challenge test is used in the diagnosis of**

    A. Dissociative amnesia

    B. Transient global amnesia

    C. Catatonia

    D. Panic disorder

    E. Endogenous depression

40. **Which of the following laboratory abnormalities is associated with malignant catatonia?**

    A. High serum magnesium

    B. Low serum iron

    C. Low liver enzymes

    D. High serum amylase

    E. Low creatinine phosphokinase

41. **All of the following indicate a better treatment response to ECT except**

    A. Shorter illness duration
    B. Past response to antidepressant treatment
    C. Significant post-ictal suppression on EEG
    D. High ictal amplitude on EEG
    E. Past history of mania

42. **While treating social anxiety disorder with SSRIs, an adequate treatment trial should probably extend to**

    A. 4 weeks
    B. 6 weeks
    C. 12 weeks
    D. 24 weeks
    E. 18 months

43. **A 32-year-old woman presents with concerns regarding her 'ugly appearance'. She had been convinced for a long time that her appearance was defective and was particularly worried about her 'streak' eyes. She admitted spending at least 14–16 hours a day thinking about her appearance and comparing herself with other people or seeking reassurance from others. Which of the following is true with regard to the treatment of this condition?**

    A. She may respond to higher than usual antidepressant doses of serotonin re-uptake inhibitors (SSRIs)
    B. There is a good evidence for response to ECT in this condition
    C. She has a comparable likelihood of response to SSRIs and non-SSRID antidepressants
    D. She will require a shorter than usual duration of treatment trial with SSRIs
    E. Cognitive behavioural therapy (CBT) has no role in the treatment

44. **A 17-year-old girl is admitted to a medical unit following a prolonged period of repeated bingeing and vomiting. She induces vomiting at least six times a day but does not use laxatives or diuretics. Which of the following laboratory finding is most likely in this patient?**

    A. Low urea levels
    B. High potassium levels
    C. Low bicarbonate levels
    D. Increased thyroxine levels
    E. High amylase levels

45. A 54-year-old African-Caribbean man had systematized persecutory delusions that prevented him from eating for 5 weeks. Following admission to a medical unit he was started on realimentation, despite which he developed diplopia, bilateral horizontal nystagmus and right sixth cranial nerve palsy. He had no past history of alcohol use. On transfer to a psychiatric ward, he was started on a normal diet but soon his phosphate levels were markedly reduced (0.26 mmol/L). The most likely diagnosis is

A. Normal pressure hydrocephalus
B. Olanzapine overdose
C. Refeeding syndrome
D. Laxative abuse
E. Hepatic failure

46. A 17-year-old girl presents with sudden-onset blindness while preparing for her school exit examinations. Which of the following suggests an ocular rather than a psychogenic cause for blindness?

A. Normal visual evoked potentials
B. Presence of tubular vision
C. Spiral changes in visual fields
D. Absence of optokinetic nystagmus
E. Disturbances in tests for proprioception

47. Which of the following culture-bound syndromes is closely associated with social phobia?

A. Brain fag syndrome in West Africa
B. Dhat syndrome in South Asia
C. Frigophobia in China
D. Taijin kyofusho in Japan
E. Arctic hysteria in Greenland

48. Which of the following mechanisms is proposed to underlie hypersalivation seen in patients taking clozapine?

A. Muscarinic M_1 blockade
B. Muscarinic M_4 stimulation
C. Histaminic H_1 blockade
E. Serotonergic $5HT_{2C}$ blockade
F. Noradrenergic α_1 blockade

49. Which of the following can increase levels of clozapine via alterations in hepatic metabolism?

A. Rifampicin
B. Phenytoin
C. Carbamazepine
D. Cigarette smoking
E. Erythromycin

50. **All of the following neuroendocrine changes are noted in depression EXCEPT**

    A. Raised salivary cortisol measures
    B. Abnormal dexamethasone suppression test
    C. Reduced Corticotropin-releasing hormone (CRH) in cerebrospinal fluid
    D. Downregulated CRH receptors
    E. Reduced adrenocorticotropic hormone (ACTH) response to CRH infusion

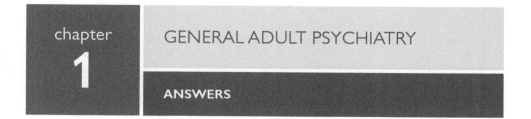
1. D.   Somatic syndrome is defined by a set of vegetative or biological features of depression. The ICD-10 criteria for somatic syndrome of depression require at least four symptoms from a list of eight. These are (1) marked loss of interest or pleasure; (2) loss of emotional reactions; (3) early-morning awakening (2 hours before normal waking time); (4) diurnal worsening of mood; (5) objective evidence of marked psychomotor retardation or agitation; (6) marked loss of appetite; (7) loss of libido and (8) 5% or more of body weight lost unintentionally in the past month. To diagnose anorexia nervosa, there must be a weight loss leading to a body weight at least 15% below the normal expected weight for age and height.

Stein G and Wilkinson G, eds. *Seminars in General Adult Psychiatry*, 2nd edn. Gaskell, 2007, p. 11.

2. C.   According to the International Pilot Study of Schizophrenia (World Health Organization 1973), 7% of 811 schizophrenia patients exhibited one or other catatonic phenomenon. Further studies that followed gave a figure of between 5% and 10%. Mannerisms are the most common catatonic phenomenon in schizophrenia, followed by stereotypies, stupor, negativism, automatism and echopraxia in order of frequency. About 10–15% of patients with catatonia meet the criteria for schizophrenia. It is widely appreciated that catatonic symptoms are more prevalent in the developing nations than in the West. When one includes all psychiatric patients, not just schizophrenia, the prevalence of catatonia increases to 10–20%. This is because depression contributes to most of the observed catatonia in practice. Immobility and mutism are the most commonly observed catatonic symptoms among depressed patients.

Hirsch SR and Weinberger DR, eds. *Schizophrenia*, 2nd edn. Blackwell Science, 2007, p.19.
Taylor MA and Fink M. Catatonia in psychiatric classification: a home of its own. *American Journal of Psychiatry* 2003; **160**: 1233–1241.

3. C.   ICD-10 clinical guidelines do not include specific criteria for SAD. However, specific criteria are included in DSM-IV (Text Revision) and the research version of ICD-10. ICD-10 provisional criteria for SAD specifies the disorder as a subtype of mood disorder where three or more episodes must occur with onset within the same 90-day period of the year for three or more consecutive years; Remissions also occur within a particular 90-day period of the year. Seasonal episodes must outnumber any non-seasonal episodes that may occur. Familial risks of affective disorders in SAD are similar to those found in non-seasonal depressive illnesses. Typical depressive symptoms of SAD respond better to bright-light therapy whereas atypical symptoms respond to phototherapy at all intensities. In phototherapy retinal light exposure is important; skin absorption is not sufficient to modify circadian rhythms or depressive symptoms. Early-morning phototherapy is superior but leads to more side-effects, such as easy startle, gastrointestinal intolerance and headaches. Conventional antidepressants have also been reported to have a therapeutic effect in SAD.

Stein G and Wilkinson G, eds. *Seminars in General Adult Psychiatry*, 2nd edn. Gaskell, 2007, p. 13.
Rodin I and Thompson C. Seasonal affective disorder. *Advances in Psychiatric Treatment*, 1997; **3**: 352–359.

4. C. Dysthymia has a 1-year prevalence of 1–3%. The lifetime prevalence according to the National Comorbidity Survey 1994 is 6%. Dysthymia has a high comorbidity with other psychiatric disorders, particularly major depression. In one series, only about 25–30% of cases were observed to occur over a lifetime in the absence of other psychiatric disorders. The comorbidity of personality disorders seems to be very high (60–80%). Early-onset dysthymia is defined as having onset before age 21.

Stein G and Wilkinson G, eds. *Seminars in General Adult Psychiatry*, 2nd edn. Gaskell, 2007, p. 14.

5. A. Follow-up studies in depression reveal two powerful predictors of recurrence: the presence of residual symptoms after apparent recovery and history of previous episodes of depression. The presence of residual symptoms increases the risk of recurrence nearly threefold, whereas past history of depression doubles the risk, with each new episode increasing the risk further. Other possible risk predictors for recurrence include somatic syndrome, reversed vegetative signs, early age of onset, and family history of mood disorders. Recurrence risk is higher in bipolar than in unipolar mood disorders.

Stein G and Wilkinson G, eds. *Seminars in General Adult Psychiatry*, 2nd edn. Gaskell, 2007, p. 17.

6. B. In community studies, 1 in 10 patients who begin with a depressive episode go on to develop an episode of mania within 10 years. If the illness begins at a younger age, the switch happens earlier. This rate increases to nearly 50% if severely depressed hospitalized patients are considered. Long-term follow-up studies blinded for severity and number of previous episodes show much lower conversion rates (3.2%). It is known that the majority of bipolar patients, particularly women, begin with depressive episodes. Among hospitalized depressed patients followed up for nearly a decade, 1% a year converted to bipolar I and 0.5% a year converted to bipolar II. However, this conversion rate is less for outpatients with depression. Factors associated with a change of polarity from unipolar to bipolar were younger age, male sex, family history of bipolarity, antidepressant-induced hypomania, hypersomnic and retarded phenomenology, psychotic depression, and a postpartum episode. The mean age at which the switch occurs is 32 years. The average number of previous episodes in those who switch varies between two and four. The huge differences in switch rates probably reflect the severity of the initial depression, the length of follow-up, and the expanding definitions of bipolar II disorder.

Angst J, et al. Diagnostic conversion from depression to bipolar disorders: results of a long-term prospective study of hospital admissions. *Journal of Affective disorders* 2005; **84**: 149–157.
Stein G and Wilkinson G, eds. *Seminars in General Adult Psychiatry*, 2nd edn. Gaskell, 2007, p. 18.

7. D. Parkes described features that may distinguish normal mourning from depression. Normal mourning is characterized by pangs of grief, angry pining, and anxiety when reminded of the loss, brief hallucinations, somatic symptoms, and identification-related behaviours. The presence of psychomotor retardation, generalized guilt and suicidal thoughts after the first month suggest development of depression.

Parkes CM and Prigerson H *Bereavement: Studies of Grief in Adult Life*, 3rd edn. Penguin, 1998.
Stein G and Wilkinson G, eds. *Seminars in General Adult Psychiatry*, 2nd edn. Gaskell, 2007, p. 19.

8. C.   Clinging behaviour and inordinate pining may be early signs of prolonged grief as described by Parkes. More recently, childhood experiences of early parental death or divorce, sudden or violent death of a loved one, and high levels of dependency on the deceased for a sense of personal well-being are thought to be associated with prolonged grief. Several of these factors suggest the role of attachment insecurity in increasing a person's vulnerability to complicated bereavement.

Lichtenthal WG, Cruess DG and Prigerson HG. A case for establishing complicated grief as a distinct mental disorder in DSM-V. *Clinical Psychology Review,* 2004; **24**: 637–662.
Stein G and Wilkinson G, eds. *Seminars in General Adult Psychiatry*, 2nd edn. Gaskell, 2007, p. 20.

9. B.   Specifiers are extensions to a diagnosis that further clarify the course, severity, or special features of the diagnosis. Note that while subtypes are mutually exclusive and jointly exhaustive patterns of diagnostic description, specifiers merely provide an opportunity to define a more homogeneous subgrouping based on observable clinical phenomenon. DSM-IV uses specifiers extensively while dealing with mood disorders. These include specifiers of the most recent episode and the longitudinal course. Specifiers of current clinical severity, psychotic features, and remission status are the most commonly used. Other descriptive specifiers include catatonic features, melancholic features, atypical features, and postpartum onset. The longitudinal course specifiers include a seasonal pattern and the presence of rapid cycling. ICD-10 does not use the term 'specifiers' separately, although the majority are discussed in the core text.

Stein G and Wilkinson G, eds. *Seminars in General Adult Psychiatry*, 2nd edn. Gaskell, 2007, p. 26.

10. C.   In any patient with bipolar disorder, the duration of individual mood episodes tends to be relatively stable throughout the course, with mania generally lasting for a shorter time than depression. But the onset may become more rapid with age. The interval from one episode to the next tends to decrease through the course of illness, although some evidence suggests a tendency for the inter-episode intervals to stabilize after approximately five episodes. Patients with seasonal patterns are more commonly of bipolar II subtype than bipolar I. The first episode is more likely to be triggered by life events than later episodes. Ambelas confirmed the strong correlation between stressful life events and first manic admissions; this association weakens as the illness progresses. This is particularly true for younger bipolar patients with mania rather than depression. This is consistent with the hypothesis of kindling phenomenon in bipolar disorders.

Stein G and Wilkinson G, eds. *Seminars in General Adult Psychiatry*, 2nd edn. Gaskell, 2007, p. 27–29.
Ambelas A. Life events and mania: a special relationship? *British Journal of Psychiatry* 1987; **150**: 235–240.

11. A.   Cushing's syndrome is very frequently, although not invariably, associated with depression. Nearly 40% of cases in one series of observation had depression whereas only 3% had mania. It is claimed that the predominance of pure depressive disorders may be a result of publication bias; controlling for this yields mixed anxiety and depression as the most common psychiatric disturbance in Cushing's syndrome. Depression in Cushing's syndrome may occur as a prodrome even before the medical disorder is diagnosed; the phenomenology may differ from primary major depression in that the symptoms are intermittent when associated with Cushing's syndrome. Psychosis occurs more commonly in association with affective states; isolated schizophreniform psychosis is rare. Delirium may occur in 15–20% of patients.

Stein G and Wilkinson G, eds. *Seminars in General Adult Psychiatry*, 2nd edn. Gaskell, 2007, p. 30.

12. C.   Lithium-related polyuria and polydipsia are seen in nearly one-third of those treated. Polyuria is usually reversible in the early stages but may become obstinate the longer the therapy lasts. When a once-daily preparation of lithium is used instead of multiple divided doses, the frequency of polyuria seems to be less, but a direct correlation between plasma peaks and polyuria is not clearly demonstrated in clinical samples. Dose reduction or use of amiloride can be tried in those who have troublesome levels of polyuria. Amiloride has relatively less propensity to cause electrolyte disturbances when co-prescribed with lithium than with other diuretics.

Stein G and Wilkinson G, eds. *Seminars in General Adult Psychiatry*, 2nd edn. Gaskell, 2007, p. 34.

13. D.   Lithium exerts minimal cardiac effects at therapeutic doses in most patients. It most commonly produces benign reversible T-wave changes (including inversion and flattening) in the resting electrocardiogram (ECG). These hypokalaemia-like changes are seen in approximately 20–30% of patients treated with lithium. ECG abnormalities of clinical significance are mainly documented at toxic levels: they include all kinds of arrhythmias (sinus node dysfunction is well documented) and QTc prolongation. SA node dysfunction is the characteristic complication of lithium therapy and can manifest clinically as sinus bradycardia or atrioventricular conduction disturbances. Other parameters such as PR and QRS intervals often remain normal. Combining carbamazepine with lithium increases the risk for cardiac arrhythmias.

Stein G and Wilkinson G, eds. *Seminars in General Adult Psychiatry*, 2nd edn. Gaskell, 2007, p. 35.
Mitchell JE and Mackenzie, TB. Cardiac effects of lithium therapy in man: a review. *J Clin Psychiatry* 1982; **43**: 47–51.

14. B.   Nearly one-fifth of lithium-treated patients show increased plasma thyroid-stimulating hormone (TSH). About 5% show thyroid enlargement (goitre) whereas 5–10% have clinical hypothyroidism. Weight gain and lethargy are the most common clinical features. These effects are dependent on dose and the duration of lithium therapy. Middle-aged women with a pre-existing propensity for hypothyroidism in the form of autoantibodies against the thyroid are the most susceptible clinical group.

Stein G and Wilkinson G, eds. *Seminars in General Adult Psychiatry*, 2nd edn. Gaskell, 2007, p. 35.

15. B.   The risk of major congenital anomalies in children exposed to lithium in the uterus is 4–12%. This is nearly three times higher than non-exposed fetuses. The UK National Teratology Information Service has concluded that lithium increases the risk of cardiac malformations by approximately eightfold. First trimester exposure to lithium increases the risk of Ebstein's anomaly by nearly 10–20 times, bringing the absolute risk to 0.05–0.1%.

Stein G and Wilkinson G, eds. *Seminars in General Adult Psychiatry*, 2nd edn. Gaskell, 2007, p. 36.
Williams K and Oke S. Lithium and pregnancy. *Psychiatric Bulletin* 2000; **24**: 229–231.

16.A. Valproate is associated with elevated plasma ammonia. In some people, hyperammonaemia may be clinically significant, resulting in hyperammonaemic encephalopathy characterized by varied clinical presentation, including irritability, agitation, drowsiness, asterixis, coma, and paradoxical seizures. Other symptoms may include loss of appetite, nausea, and vomiting. Valproic acid-induced hyperammonaemic encephalopathy may occur in people with normal liver function, despite normal doses and serum levels. It is more common in children with urea cycle enzyme deficiencies. Other risk factors include concomitant antiepileptic prescriptions (especially topiramate), underlying liver disease or hypoalbuminaemia, initiation of high-dose and long-term therapy. Propionate, a metabolite of valproate reduces the hepatic *N*-acetylglutamate concentration, which is an obligatory activator of carbamoyl phosphate synthetase 1 (CPS-1), the first enzyme of the urea cycle. Another potential mechanism may be via valproate-induced reduction in hepatic carnitine levels.

Stein G and Wilkinson G, eds. *Seminars in General Adult Psychiatry*, 2nd edn. Gaskell, 2007, p. 38. Barrueto F Jr and Hack JB. Hyperammonemia and coma without hepatic dysfunction induced by valproate therapy. *Academic Emergency Medicine* 2001; **8**: 999–1001.

17. C. Nausea, ataxia, and dizziness are common side-effects of carbamazepine; usually, none of these in isolation warrants a cessation of therapy. A maculopapular rash is noted in nearly 1 in 10 patients receiving carbamazepine. This usually occurs within 2 weeks of therapy and often requires cessation of treatment if associated with an abnormal blood count. Although leucopenia is seen in 1–2% of patients, serious agranulocytosis occurs rarely (about eight per million prescriptions). This bone marrow toxicity warrants a cessation of therapy and is indicated by a total white blood cell (WBC) count of less than 3000 per mm^3 or a neutrophil count less than 1500 per mm^3. Hyponatraemia is a common side-effect but levels up to 125 mEq/L can be managed conservatively without requiring sudden cessation of treatment. Elevation of thyroid-stimulating hormone does not necessitate stopping carbamazepine.

Stein G and Wilkinson G, eds. *Seminars in General Adult Psychiatry*, 2nd edn. Gaskell, 2007, p. 39.

18. D. Various clinical, biological, and genetic factors that predict lithium responsiveness in prophylaxis of bipolar disorder have been studied. The presence of typical features of bipolar disorder, good inter-episode clinical recovery, a family history of bipolar disorder, experiencing mania as the first bipolar episode, and a good response to lithium in the acute manic phase predict lithium responsiveness. The presence of neurological signs, comorbid substance use, and the presence of rapid cycling predict a poor response to lithium. The lithium response in a sample composed of relatives of lithium responder probands was 67% compared with 30% in the control group; this indicates that lithium responsiveness may have a certain degree of heritability.

Stein G and Wilkinson G, eds. *Seminars in General Adult Psychiatry*, 2nd edn. Gaskell, 2007, p. 40. Grof P, Duffy A, Cavazzoni P, et al. Is response to prophylactic lithium a familial trait? *Journal of Clinical Psychiatry* 2002; **63**: 942–947.

19. C. Parental divorce between birth and age 7, regardless of subsequent remarriage, was predictive of a twofold higher depression risk. The relative risk of depression was highest for children whose single parent remarried into a conflictual relationship following divorce. It was shown that the quality of parental relationship, especially in relation to continuing conflict among those taking parental responsibilities, has a major effect on the subsequent risk of depression. Although childhood socioeconomic status was found to be a significant predictor of later depression, the risk for depression associated with parental divorce was found to be of a similar magnitude across categories of childhood socioeconomic status. There is little evidence that childhood bereavement itself predisposes to adult depression.

Stein G and Wilkinson G, eds. *Seminars in General Adult Psychiatry*, 2nd edn. Gaskell, 2007, p. 54.
Gilman SE, *et al*. Family disruption in childhood and risk of adult depression. *American Journal of Psychiatry* 2003; **160**: 939–946.

20. E. Only 30% of those with depression give no history of significant life events. Depression itself may generate negative life events (reverse causality). Similarly, there may be a genetic contribution to the experience of adverse life events, making the gene–environment interaction more complex. The Life Events and Difficulties Scale is considered to be the standard life events assessment instrument. This scale is based on contextual measurement of the threat posed by life events (i.e. an event can be considered as significant only in accordance with social and cultural backgrounds and the life situation in which it occurs). It is shown that suicide attempters have a higher rate of life events than those with depression. Loss, humiliation, or separation events highly correlate with depression.

Stein G and Wilkinson G, eds. *Seminars in General Adult Psychiatry*, 2nd edn. Gaskell, 2007, p. 55.

21. C. If negative events are ascribed to external, unstable, and specific causes, one may come to believe that they are modifiable; this will also induce less self-blame and guilt and will not induce feelings of helplessness or hopelessness. In contrast, individuals whose locus of control for negative events is internal, global, and non-specific show a higher degree of self-blame and depression-prone attitude. These individuals possess a high degree of information-processing biases characterized by the perception of a higher than possible probability for aversive events and belief that such events are uncontrollable (fatalistic). They also have a fragile self-esteem.

Stein G and Wilkinson G, eds. *Seminars in General Adult Psychiatry*, 2nd edn. Gaskell, 2007, p. 58.

22. A. Rimonabant was approved in Europe as an anti-obesity agent in 2006. Rimonabant is a selective antagonist of the cannabinoid type 1 receptor, and it is the first member of a new class of compounds that targets the endocannabinoid system. But concerns have been raised regarding the psychiatric adverse effects of this drug. A meta-analysis by the American Food and Drug Administration showed that 26% of people given rimonabant 20 mg versus 14% of those given placebo had a psychiatric symptom reported as an adverse event. The side-effects range from depressed mood to anxiety and often led to co-prescription of a psychotropic or withdrawal of the drug. The relative risk for psychiatric adverse events in the rimonabant group was twice higher than the placebo group.

Christensen R, *et al*. Efficacy and safety of the weight-loss drug rimonabant: a meta-analysis of randomised trials. *Lancet* 2007; **370**: 1706–1713.

23. D.   Kapur proposed that in the normal individual, the role of mesolimbic dopamine is to attach significance or 'salience' to an external stimulus or an internal thought. This converts a neutral piece of information into attention-grabbing information. In acute psychosis where a hyperdopaminergic state is noted in the mesolimbic system, insignificant events and perceptions receive inappropriate salience. For example, an innocuous smile of a stranger may be given a high degree of 'aberrant salience' leading to delusional elaborations. On a similar note, when such aberrant salience is attached to internally generated self-speech, hallucinations may be experienced. Antipsychotics are claimed to 'dampen the salience' of these abnormal experiences rather than erase the symptoms, and provide the platform for a process of psychological resolution.

Murray R, *et al.*, eds. *Essential Psychiatry*, 4th edn. Cambridge University Press, 2008, p. 302.
Kapur, S. Psychosis as a state of aberrant salience: a framework linking biology, phenomenology, and pharmacology in schizophrenia. *American Journal of Psychiatry* 2003; **160**: 13–23.

24. C.   DSM-IV-TR research criteria require both severe muscle rigidity and elevated temperature to be present following recent administration of an antipsychotic. In addition, at least two associated signs, symptoms, or laboratory findings must be present. The associated symptoms listed in DSM research criteria include diaphoresis, dysphagia, tremors, incontinence, mutism, tachycardia, elevated blood pressure, leucocytosis, changes in the level of consciousness, and laboratory evidence of muscle injury. NMS must be distinguished from serotonin syndrome. NMS is an idiosyncratic reaction to therapeutic dosages of neuroleptic agents, whereas serotonin syndrome is a toxic reaction due to overstimulation of 5-HT_{2a} receptors; distinguishing features include bradykinesia and lead pipe rigidity in NMS, whereas hyperkinesia and myoclonus are evident in serotonin syndrome.

Kay J and Tasman A. *Essentials of Psychiatry*. John Wiley and Sons, 2006, p. 833.

25. A.   Nocturnal panic refers to waking from sleep with an abrupt and discrete sense of intense fear accompanied by cognitive and physical symptoms of arousal. It does not differ significantly from panic attacks that occur during wakeful states. Most patients with nocturnal panic experience panic attacks during wakeful states too. But a small subset with predominantly circumscribed nocturnal panic has been described. Most patients report that nocturnal panic occurs between 1 and 3 hours after sleep onset. It is a non-REM event, usually occurring in late Stage II or early Stage III sleep. It is not accompanied by any electroencephalographic abnormalities.

Kay J and Tasman A. *Essentials of Psychiatry*. John Wiley and Sons, 2006, p. 750.
Craske M and Tsao J. Assessment and treatment of nocturnal panic attacks. *Sleep Medicine Reviews* 2005; **9**: 173–184.

26. B.   Disrupted sleep architecture is a long-recognized feature of mood disorders. Several sleep-related electroencephalogram (EEG) changes have been noted in around 90% of those with depression. Short REM latency, increased amount of REM sleep, increased REM density, especially in the first REM episode, prolonged sleep latency, increased frequency of awakenings with low arousal threshold, reduced slow-wave sleep, and shifting of delta sleep to second-stage NREM sleep are some of the notable changes. Some reports have suggested that bipolar depression may be atypical with respect to sleep changes in that daytime sleepiness and increased sleep efficiency are reported. In hypomania/mania, short REM latency, inability to fall asleep, short sleep duration, and reduced delta sleep are seen. In patients who have secondary depression due to a chronic medical condition, REM sleep may be reduced.

Kay J and Tasman A. *Essentials of Psychiatry*. John Wiley and Sons, 2006, p. 750.

27. C. Normally REM sleep is associated with loss of muscle tone (atonia) and dreaming. In some patients, as an isolated condition or as a prodrome for later neurodegenerative disorders such as Lewy body dementia/Parkinson's disease, this normal atonia is absent. This then leads to 'dreams being acted out' with uncontrolled limb movements. This is called REM sleep behavioural disorder. Patients can recall dreams when awakened, unlike sleep terror. The behaviours may be more complex than simple sleepwalking. Periodic limb movement disorder is characterized by periodic episodes of repetitive and stereotyped limb movements that occur during sleep. These movements can cause clinical sleep disturbance expressed by insomnia or excessive daytime sleepiness. This is not a dream-related behaviour, unlike REM sleep behavioural disorder. Restless legs syndrome, in simplistic terms, is the daytime extension of periodic limb movement disorder wherein episodic akathisia and motor restlessness are seen during the day and at night.

Kay J and Tasman A. *Essentials of Psychiatry*. John Wiley and Sons, 2006, p. 748.

28. D. Pharmacological treatment options for restless leg syndrome include dopaminergic agents (L-dopa, pergolide, pramipexole), anticonvulsants (gabapentin, carbamazepine), certain opioid drugs, and clonazepam. Amitriptyline has no role in the management of restless leg syndrome. An increase in periodic limb movements observed during sleep has been reported as a side-effect of tricyclics. Some patients may report new-onset restless leg syndrome in association with SSRIs or tricyclics when treated for depression.

Kay J and Tasman A. *Essentials of Psychiatry*. John Wiley and Sons, 2006, p. 747.

29. A. It is important to realize that clear-cut demarcations between psychogenic or organic erectile dysfunctions are difficult to ascertain in clinical practice. But certain clues that may favour a psychogenic origin/overlay of erectile dysfunction include sudden onset of the problem, early collapse of erection (as against complete absence of tumescence), preserved spontaneous (early morning) and self-stimulated erections, antecedent (temporally related) problems or changes in relationship, a history of significant preceding or ongoing life events, and evidence of psychological problems. Clues that may indicate an organic aetiology include preserved ejaculation in spite of impaired erection, unperturbed libido (in the early stages), and a history of antecedent physical injury, surgeries, or vascular risk factors in the medical history, smoking, and other prescribed or recreational drug use.

Lue TF. Erectile dysfunction. *New England Journal of Medicine* 2000; **342**: 1802–1813.

30. D. Apomorphine is a dopamine receptor agonist which stimulates both dopamine D1 and D2 receptors and is sometimes used in male erectile dysfunction. Phosphodiesterase-5 (PDE-5) is an enzyme found in the trabecular smooth muscle of the penis. It catalyses the degradation of cGMP, which results in an elevated cytosolic calcium concentration and muscular contraction leading to erection. PDE-5 inhibitors such as sildenafil, vardenafil, and tadalafil block this biochemical pathway to promote erection. Sildenafil and vardenafil must be taken 1 hour before sexual activity to enable their action. Alprostadil is prostaglandin E_1, which causes smooth muscle relaxation and subsequent vasodilation by acting on adenylate cyclase to increase the intracellular cyclic adenosine monophosphate (cAMP) concentration. Yohimbine is not commonly used for erectile dysfunction; it is an adrenergic antagonist relatively selective for alpha-2 receptors. The site of action of yohimbine when used for erectile dysfunction is suspected to be central rather than peripheral as the predominant subtype of alpha-adrenoceptor in penile erectile tissue is alpha-1 type rather than alpha-2 type.

Stein G and Wilkinson G, eds. *Seminars in General Adult Psychiatry*, 2nd edn. Gaskell, 2007, p. 682.

31. C. Not everyone who experiences a traumatic event goes on to develop PTSD. It is difficult to predict exactly who will go on to develop PTSD. Two factors most associated with future risk of PTSD in those exposed to trauma are perceived lack of social support and peri-traumatic dissociation. The possibility of predicting PTSD has led to designing of predictive screening instruments to be used shortly after a traumatic event. The 10-item Trauma Screening Questionnaire (TSQ) is one of the best validated. The TSQ is a predictive screening instrument for victims of violent crime 1–3 weeks after the assault. In spite of high rates of sensitivity and specificity, a lower positive predictive value (around 0.48) means that although the TSQ can detect the vast majority of PTSD sufferers at 1 month, 50% of those who screened positive will not develop PTSD. Other scales listed in the question are not used directly for predicting PTSD. The Holmes and Rahe Social Adjustment Scale is used to measure the impact of life events by means of arbitrary values attached to different types of common life events. The Life Events and Difficulties scale is used to measure the contextual threat posed by life events. Appraisal of the Life Events Scale is designed to provide an index of the three primary appraisal dimensions (threat, challenge, and loss) described in Lazarus and Folkman's transactional model of stress. The Abbreviated Injury Scale is an anatomical scoring system used to classify motor accident victims to enable emergency physical interventions.

Walters JTR, Bisson JI and Shepherd JP. Predicting posttraumatic stress disorder: validation of the Trauma Screening Questionnaire in victims of assault. *Psychological Medicine* 2007; **37**: 143–150.

32. C. Niacin (nicotinic acid) is a water-soluble vitamin used as a drug for hyperlipidaemia. It can induce a visible skin flush response that is caused by prostaglandin-mediated cutaneous vasodilatation. This normal flush response is reduced in patients with schizophrenia. The use of niacin challenge as a simple biochemical test for schizophrenia has been proposed. Depending on the criteria used, the prevalence rates of attenuated or absent response to a niacin skin patch in patients with schizophrenia ranged from 49% to 90%, compared with 8% to 23% in healthy control subjects. This abnormal flush response has also been reported in first-degree relatives of schizophrenia patients. The estimated heritability ranges from 47% to 54%. The attenuated flush response to a niacin patch seen in schizophrenia patients was not observed in patients with depression, bipolar disorder or autism. The reduced niacin flush response in patients with schizophrenia was not affected by medication status, antipsychotic drug doses, or substances such as cigarette, coffee, or alcohol consumption.

Chang S, *et al.* Impaired flush response to niacin skin patch among schizophrenia patients and their nonpsychotic relatives: the effect of genetic loading. *Schizophrenia Bulletin* 2009; **35**: 213–221.

33. A. Tryptophan depletion is used as an intervention to deplete serotonin (5-HT) in humans. It is noted to reverse the antidepressant effects of SSRIs and monoamine oxidase inhibitors (MAOIs) in patients in remission with a history of depression but not in patients treated with antidepressants that promote catecholaminergic rather than serotonergic neurotransmission (such as tricyclic antidepressants, reboxetine, or buproprion). Patients who are either unmedicated and/or fully remitted are much less likely to experience relapse than patients who are recently medicated and partially remitted. Recently remitted patients who have been treated with non-pharmacological therapies such as total sleep deprivation, electroconvulsive therapy, or phototherapy and possibly CBT do not commonly show full clinical relapse with tryptophan depletion.

Stein G and Wilkinson G, eds. *Seminars in General Adult Psychiatry*, 2nd edn. Gaskell, 2007, p. 64. O'Reardon JP, *et al.* Response to tryptophan depletion in major depression treated with either cognitive therapy or selective serotonin reuptake inhibitor antidepressants. *Biological Psychiatry* 2004; **55**: 957–959.

34. B. An increased density of $5HT_2$ binding sites has been shown in post-mortem studies of depressed/suicidal patients. The increase in $5HT_{2A}$ receptors is most prominent in the dorsolateral prefrontal cortex and in platelets of medication naïve patients. A *reduction* in $5HT_{1A}$ receptors has also been noted in the cortex. In contrast, long-term antidepressant treatment has been shown to reduce $5HT_2$ receptors and increase $5HT_{1A}$ function. But these changes may not be causative in antidepressant action as they pre-date any clinical response in those who have started antidepressant therapy. Of note, ECT treatment actually increases $5HT_{2A}$ receptors. Most directly acting $5HT_{1A}$ agonists have poor antidepressant activity. Chronic antidepressant treatment induces a reduction in β adrenoreceptor density around 2 weeks after starting antidepressants; this correlates with therapeutic effects. Unmedicated suicide victims show a greater density of β adrenoreceptors.

Stein G and Wilkinson G, eds. *Seminars in General Adult Psychiatry*, 2nd edn. Gaskell, 2007, p. 64–65.

35. D. The severity of lithium toxicity has a feeble relationship, if any, with levels of serum lithium. Neurotoxicity can occur even within therapeutic levels of lithium. The symptoms of lithium toxicity can be grouped into gastrointestinal symptoms such as nausea, diarrhoea, vomiting; neurological symptoms such as severe tremors (coarse), cerebellar ataxia, slurred speech, myoclonus, and spasticity; mental symptoms such as drowsiness, disorientation, and apathy. Most patients make a full recovery when lithium is stopped but serum levels may continue to rise due to intracellular lithium release even after cessation of treatment. Rarely, persistent cerebellar damage and cognitive impairment are reported following lithium toxicity.

Stein G and Wilkinson G, eds. *Seminars in General Adult Psychiatry*, 2nd edn. Gaskell, 2007, p. 37.

36. A. Amitriptyline has the highest affinity for central muscarinic acetylcholine receptors among various antidepressants. Its affinity is nearly one-tenth of the affinity shown by atropine. This is followed by protriptyline and clomipramine. Trazodone has very low muscarinic affinity. Anticholinergic side-effects of tricyclics include dry mouth, blurred vision, urinary retention, constipation, memory impairment, and confusion especially in elderly people.

Stein G and Wilkinson G, eds. *Seminars in General Adult Psychiatry*, 2nd edn. Gaskell, 2007, p. 85.

37. D. One in every 100 000 patients treated with monoamine oxidase inhibitors such as tranylcypromine die due to fatal hypertensive reaction. The fatality rate can also be expressed as 1 in every 8000 hypertensive reactions. The so-called 'cheese reaction' is mainly characterized by skin flushing, tachycardia, dyspnoea, sweating, hypertension, conjunctival injection, and headache. The reaction is usually self-limiting, with signs and symptoms lasting from few minutes to a few hours. Tyramine is formed by the decarboxylation of the amino acid tyrosine; it is mainly catabolized via oxidation by monoamine oxidase-A (MAO-A) in man. Thus MAO-A acts as a protective barrier against high tyramine levels in the nervous system. Unmetabolized tyramine is transported into adrenergic nerve terminals where it displaces noradrenaline, causing hypertension.

Stein G and Wilkinson G, eds. *Seminars in General Adult Psychiatry*, 2nd edn. Gaskell, 2007, p. 91.

38. C.   Data from the Office of National Statistics from 1993–2002 have demonstrated a significantly higher rate of fatal overdose (fatal toxicity index) with the antidepressant venlafaxine than with SSRIs. Venlafaxine has a similar lethality to TCAs in cases of overdose; most deaths are ascribed to cardiac effects of the drug. Overall, approximately 10% of venlafaxine overdoses that are reported have proven fatal. Blood pressure increases are common in therapeutic doses but severe increases do not appear to be a significant feature of overdose. Fatal toxicity indices (FTIs) are calculated using recorded deaths attributed to drug overdose obtained from prescribing data. TCAs (in particular dothiepin) have been associated with a higher FTI than venlafaxine, which in turn has been associated with a higher FTI than SSRIs.

Medicines and Healthcare Products Regulatory Agency. Updated prescribing advice for venlafaxine Effexor/Effexor XL (Accessed 28 December 2008 www.mhra.gov.uk).
Stein G and Wilkinson G, eds. *Seminars in General Adult Psychiatry*, 2nd edn. Gaskell, 2007, p. 95.

39. C.   In the 'lorazepam challenge test' (coined by George Bidder), an intravenous line is established and a syringe containing 2–4 mg of lorazepam in 2 mL of solution is prepared, and 1 mg is injected. In the next 2–5 minutes if no reduction is observed in catatonic features, the second 1 mg of lorazepam is injected, and the assessment is repeated. It is noted that more than 80% of patients with catatonia have a rapid reduction in symptoms with an intravenous lorazepam challenge. Such a response to lorazepam typically results in a lorazepam treatment trial, followed by electroconvulsive therapy if substantial relief is not maintained. Fink and Taylor suggest that adhering to this algorithm achieves remission of catatonia in almost all patients. Amytal interview using intravenous barbiturates/benzodiazepines has been used in dissociative amnesia/fugue.

Bush G, *et al*. Catatonia, II: treatment with lorazepam and electroconvulsive therapy. *Acta Psychiatrica Scandinavica* 1996; **93**: 137–143.
Fink M and Taylor MA. Catatonia: subtype or syndrome in DSM? *American Journal of Psychiatry* 2006; **163**: 1875–1876.

40. B.   The syndrome of malignant catatonia is severe form of catatonia characterized by fever, muscle rigidity and autonomic instability and can be fatal (through renal failure, pulmonary embolism or arrhythmias) if not treated promptly. It is indistinguishable from neuroleptic malignant syndrome. ECT is the treatment of choice. Laboratory studies often help to assess the overall health of a catatonic patient; they rarely help in identifying the cause or confirm the diagnosis of catatonia in isolation. Elevated levels of creatinine phosphokinase (CPK), elevated liver enzymes, and leucocytosis are some of the changes noted in patients with malignant catatonia. Low serum iron levels are associated with malignant catatonia; it is also observed in some patients with neuroleptic malignant syndrome. Serum calcium and magnesium levels are either normal or low in catatonia.

Ananth J, *et al*. Neuroleptic malignant syndrome: risk factors, pathophysiology, and treatment. *Acta Neuropsychiatrica* 2004; **16**: 219–228.

41. E. Medication resistance and chronicity of depression are two often noted factors that predict lower response rates to ECT. Though ECT can provide significant benefit for patients who are resistant to medication, the degree of response may be less than in depressed patients who are not considered to have such resistance. Similarly, patients with longer durations of continuous depressive illness are less likely to respond to ECT. Post-ictal suppression and ictal amplitude are two main EEG-related features during ECT treatment that are associated with positive efficacy. Post-ictal suppression refers to the acute fall in EEG amplitude immediately after the ECT-induced seizure terminates. Ictal EEG amplitude or power measured as voltage is felt to be related to seizure strength or intensity. Bipolar depression does not respond to ECT differently from unipolar depression when other variables are controlled for.

Tyrer P and Silk K, eds. *Cambridge Textbook of Effective Treatments in Psychiatry*. Cambridge University Press, 2008, p. 62.
Daly JJ, *et al*. ECT in bipolar and unipolar depression: differences in speed of response. *Bipolar Disorders* 2001; **3**: 95–104.

42. C. SSRIs are now widely used as first-line agents in social anxiety disorder – both limited and generalized subtypes. An adequate trial of treatment with SSRIs in social anxiety must extend to 12 weeks, with a minimum of 6–8 weeks at the highest tolerated doses administered before considering a switch. It may take many months to consolidate a full treatment response and achieve a full remission. If the treatment is effective, it is recommended that it be continued for at least for a year, and then very gradually tapered off.

Murray R, *et al*, eds. *Essential Psychiatry*, 4th edn. Cambridge University Press, 2008, p. 158.
Ballenger JC, *et al*. Consensus statement on social anxiety disorder from the International Consensus Group on Depression and Anxiety. *Journal of Clinical Psychiatry* 1998; **59**: 54–60.

43. A. The amount of evidence for treatment of body dysmorphic disorder (BDD) is limited, but it is accepted that serotonin reuptake inhibitors (SSRIs) and cognitive–behavioural therapy (CBT) are the treatments of choice. Antidepressants, antipsychotics, or electroconvulsive therapy are not efficacious for BDD, even though the data are limited. BDD symptoms of delusional patients appear as likely as symptoms of non-delusional patients to respond to an SSRI. SSRIs improve preoccupations, distress, and insight with an associated reduction in BDD-related behaviours such as mirror-checking, etc. The patient need not have depression to experience the beneficial effect. Although data are limited with respect to dose-finding studies, it is accepted that BDD often requires higher SSRI doses than those typically used in the treatment of depression, with variable response times ranging from 4–5 weeks to 9 weeks. Many patients may thus require longer than the usual treatment trial.

Phillips KA. Pharmacologic treatment of body dysmorphic disorder: review of the evidence and a recommended treatment approach. *CNS Spectrums* 2002; **7**: 453–60.

44. E. Elevations of serum amylase have been reported in 25–60% of anorexic/bulimic patients who repeatedly vomit. This amylase appears to derive from the salivary fraction and not the pancreas. Thus it may be associated with a clinical finding of parotid gland enlargement. The use of serum amylase measurement as an index of clinical symptomatology in eating disorders is currently limited as the correlation between amylase levels and symptom severity is poor. Low urea levels are seen in restricting the type of anorexia; they may be increased in those who vomit repeatedly. Hypokalaemia is a feature of laxative abuse or repeated vomiting in anorexia. High bicarbonate levels are associated with vomiting whereas low levels are seen in laxative abuse. Thyroid hormone (T3) is reduced in anorexia; basal TSH values and thyroxine levels may be normal (low T3 syndrome).

Stein G and Wilkinson G, eds. *Seminars in General Adult Psychiatry*, 2nd edn. Gaskell, 2007, p. 621.
Fairburn CG and Harrison PJ. Eating disorders. *Lancet* 2003; **361**: 407–416.

45. C. Refeeding syndrome refers to severe electrolyte and fluid shift associated with metabolic abnormalities in patients with malnutrition undergoing realimentation. Refeeding syndrome can occur in people with eating disorders and alcoholism but it is often missed in psychiatric units. This patient has developed features of low phosphate and thiamine deficiency following realimentation. The clinical features are related to the shift in metabolism that occurs on refeeding. A change from fat to carbohydrate-based energy production occurs. A glucose load stimulates insulin release, causing increased cellular uptake of glucose, phosphate, potassium, magnesium, and water. This will result in hypophosphataemia, which in turn may cause a deficit in adenosine triphosphate (ATP) with widespread neuromuscular and haematolgical consequences. Thiamine deficiency occurs due to increased cellular utilization of thiamine in response to carbohydrate refeeding and is associated with the precipitation of Wernicke's encephalopathy.

Catani, M and Howells, R. Risks and pitfalls for the management of refeeding syndrome in psychiatric patients. *Psychiatric Bulletin* 2007; **31**: 209–211.

46. D. Non-organic visual loss may be psychogenic (conversion phenomenon) or secondary to malingering. It is more common among younger age groups and females, with the most frequently reported complaints being a reduction of visual acuity with or without loss of field. Absence of underlying optic nerve pathology is suggested by the demonstration of normal evoked potentials. On visual field testing the patients may have an inconsistent spiral field. When the patient acknowledges sighting the stimulus at some point on a horizontal axis, the examiner then moves around the field in a circle (clockwise or anticlockwise). This will produce a progressively constricting field and when the same horizontal axis is reached again, the stimulus will only be sighted at a much closer point to the centre. Some patients may have tubular vision. In the presence of true visual field loss, the area of constricted field expands with increasing distance of the testing screen. In non-organic visual loss such field defects remain unchanged in width when tangent screen testing is performed at varying distances. This produces what is known as 'tubular fields'. Simple tests of proprioception such as the finger–nose test are easily performed by blind patients; in non-organic visual loss, patients may be incapable of carrying out these tests. Intact vision (acuity at least 6/60) will elicit a positive optokinetic nystagmus (eyes moving with a black/white striped drum rolling in front of the eyes). The absence of such nystagmus indicates an ocular rather than psychogenic cause for visual loss.

Beatty S. Psychogenic medicine: Non-organic visual loss. *Postgraduate Medical Journal* 1999; **75**: 201–207.

47. D. Taijin Kyofusho (or anthropophobia: a fear of interpersonal relationships) could be considered as a cultural expression of social phobia among Japanese. Hikikomori, manifest by complete withdrawal from social life, is very closely related. Patients show severe obsession and fear of social contact with extreme self-consciousness regarding appearance, blushing, stuttering, or emitting offensive odours. Brain fag syndrome (known as studiation madness in the Caribbean) is characterized by variety of medically unexplained somatic symptoms, anxiety, depression, and fatigue. Symptoms may be triggered by the effort of reading; it is seen in students from a West African background. Dhat syndrome is characterized by complaints of discharge of semen in urine with no urological cause; this may be associated with fatigue and anxiety of loss of fertility and reproductive potency. Frigophobia (Pa-Leng) is a chronic anxiety state with phobia for cold; the patients may dress compulsively in heavy clothes and may become housebound for the fear of 'cold attack'. Arctic hysteria or Piboloktoq is an acute dissociative episode of disruptive behaviour characterized by an irritable prodromal period and subsequent wild, excited, and risky behaviour.

Stein G and Wilkinson G, eds. *Seminars in General Adult Psychiatry*, 2nd edn. Gaskell, 2007, p. 806.

48. B.   Both muscarinic M3 and M4 receptors are expressed in salivary glands. In general, stimulation of these receptors leads to increased salivation. Clozapine has antagonistic properties at muscarinic receptors (M1 to M3, and M5) but acts as an agonist at the M4 receptor. Olanzapine also has direct M4-agonistic properties and can produce hypersalivation; pirenzepine, an M4 antagonist, alleviates hypersalivation. In addition, clozapine may exacerbate salivation through its alpha-2 antagonism.

Stein G and Wilkinson G, eds. *Seminars in General Adult Psychiatry*, 2nd edn. Gaskell, 2007, p. 255.

49. E.   Clozapine is mostly metabolized via the CYP1A2, 3A4, and 2C19 enzymes. Cigarette smoking and caffeine induce CYP1A2; this can reduce clozapine levels in plasma. Rifampicin, carbamazepine, and phenytoin induce CYP3A4 and thus reduce clozapine levels. Erythromycin inhibits CYP3A4 and ciprofloxacin inhibits CYP1A2; both increase clozapine levels.

Stein G and Wilkinson G, eds. *Seminars in General Adult Psychiatry*, 2nd edn. Gaskell, 2007, p. 254.

50. C.   Depression is associated with many neuroendocrine changes in hypothalamic-pituitary-adrenal cortex axis. Raised cortisol (measured in blood or saliva), abnormal dexamethasone suppression test (non-suppression of cortisol levels after overnight dexamethasone administration), and abnormal dexamethasone–corticotrophin releasing hormone (CRH) response (mediated via reduced ACTH response to CRH infusion), raised CRH levels in cerebrospinal fluid and down regulated CRH receptors are some of the reported changes.

Murray R, et al, eds. *Essential Psychiatry*, 4th edn. Cambridge University Press, 2008, p. 268.

FORENSIC AND REHABILITATION PSYCHIATRY

1. **Which of the following is true with regard to the association between schizophrenia and recorded crime rates?**
   A. The risk is increased for non-violent crimes only
   B. The risk is increased for violent but not non-violent crimes
   C. The risk of crime is increased for narrow diagnosis of schizophrenia rather than broad diagnosis of psychosis
   D. The association is seen only for less serious violent acts
   E. The risk is highest for violent crimes for both narrowly defined schizophrenia and broadly defined psychosis

2. **All of the following factors are significantly associated with increased risk of violence among those with schizophrenia except**
   A. Comorbid substance use
   B. Comorbid personality disorder
   C. Acute psychotic symptoms
   D. Non-compliance with treatment
   E. Comorbid depression

3. **Which of the following is true about the epidemiology of violence in schizophrenia?**
   A. Most offenders with schizophrenia offend for the first time after the onset of illness
   B. Most offenders with schizophrenia have delusions directly relevant to violence
   C. Most offenders with schizophrenia do not have substance use problems
   D. Most offenders with schizophrenia do not reoffend if the illness is diagnosed
   E. The risk factors increasing violence is similar in both schizophrenia and non-schizophrenia populations

4. **The amount of societal violence rate that can be ascribed to psychiatric illness is**
   A. 1 in 10
   B. 1 in 20
   C. 1 in 5
   D. 1 in 2
   E. 1 in 100

5. **With respect to population-attributable risk of violence in those with schizophrenia, which of the following is true?**

    A. It is a more important public health measure than relative risk
    B. It increases with increasing overall crime rates
    C. Most crimes in Europe are committed by those with schizophrenia
    D. It decreases with increasing overall crime rates
    E. It represents the amount of crime that would remain if schizophrenia is completely eliminated from a population

6. **The term filicide refers to**

    A. Killing of father by son
    B. Killing of a sister by another
    C. Killing of husband by wife
    D. Killing of a child by mother
    E. Killing of a parent by child

7. **To be applied successfully the fitness to plead criteria must be found relevant to a defendant at the time of**

    A. The criminal offence
    B. The trial proceedings
    C. Being interviewed in custody
    D. Sentenced imprisonment
    E. The arrest

8. **Which of the following refers to assessment of medical negligence?**

    A. McNaughton's criteria
    B. MacArthur's competency assessment tool
    C. Pritchard's criteria
    D. Hare's checklist
    E. Bolam criteria

9. **A 'trial of facts' takes place in which of the following conditions?**

    A. Defendant is highly suggestible
    B. Defendant is unfit to plead
    C. Defendant has learning disability
    D. Defendant has amnesia for the event of crime
    E. Defendant is found not guilty by reason of insanity

10. **Which of the following is a structured clinical risk assessment tool used in a forensic setting?**

    A. Psychopathy Check List – Revised
    B. Violence Risk Appraisal Guide (VRAG)
    C. Iterative classification tree
    D. HCR-20
    E. Minnesota Multiphasic Personality Inventory (MMPI)

11. **Which of the following is true with regard to VRAG?**

A. It incorporates HCR-20 as a subscale

B. It contains 24 items

C. Presence of schizophrenia is a predictor of lower risk

D. Psychopathy is not included as a predictor

E. It is a structured clinical risk assessment tool

12. **Which of the following is true with regard to the association between learning disability and offending?**

A. Above average IQ is an independent risk factor for offending

B. Severity of learning disability correlates with severity of the offence

C. Degree of learning disability correlates with rate of offending

D. Homicide is the most common offence committed by those with a learning disability

E. Substance abuse is associated with a risk of offending among the learning disabled

13. **The proportion of male remand prisoners in England and Wales with at least one personality disorder is**

A. 20%

B. 10%

C. 50%

D. 33%

E. 80%

14. **The McNaughton rules are often discussed when a defence of insanity is used. Which of the following is NOT a factor that can be used for the insanity defence under the McNaughton rules?**

A. Disease of the mind

B. Defect of reason

C. Not knowing the nature and quality of the act

D. Defect of moral judgement

E. Absence of knowledge that the act is wrong

15. **Which of the following statements is true with regard to the relationship between antisocial personality disorder and psychopathy?**

A. A minor subgroup of those with psychopathy have anti-social personality disorder

B. All those with antisocial personality are psychopathic

C. Only multiple homicide offenders can be classified as psychopathic

D. Antisocial personality is a better predictor of violence risk than psychopathy

E. Impulsive aggression is more common in those with antisocial personality without psychopathy

16. **Various neurobiological abnormalities have been documented in those with psychopathy. Which of the following is one such feature?**

A. Reduced fear-based learning
B. Increased baseline autonomic arousal
C. Reduced verbal IQ
D. Increased reactive autonomic arousal on stimulation
E. Increased P300 differentiation between target and non-target stimuli

17. **Which of the following is associated with a risk of aggression or violent behaviour in those without serious mental illness?**

A. Neurological soft signs
B. Executive function deficits
C. Minor physical anomalies
D. Obstetric complications in pregnancy
E. All of the above

18. **In those who experience childhood maltreatment which of the following has been associated with a later risk of antisocial behaviour?**

A. Serotonin transporter polymorphism
B. MAO enzyme polymorphism
C. Dopamine receptor polymorphism
D. COMT polymorphism
E. Trinucleotide repeats in chromosome X

19. **The most common group of mental disorders diagnosed among homicide offenders is**

A. Personality disorders
B. Substance use disorders
C. Schizophreniform disorders
D. Affective disorders
E. Learning disabilities

20. **The proportion of those who commit homicide who are in contact with mental health services within the previous year is**

A. 1–4%
B. 8–11%
C. 40–43%
D. 60–63%
E. 80–86%

21. **Compared with homicide perpetrators who kill those who are known to them, perpetrators who kill strangers are more likely to**

A. Have a history of mental disorder
B. Have a history of contact with mental health services
C. Be a young female
D. Have psychiatric symptoms at the time of offence
E. Have a history of drug misuse

22. **Which of the following is true with regard to men convicted of a sexual offence compared with men with no history of sexual offences in the general population?**
    A. Sexual offenders have a similar risk for psychiatric hospitalization
    B. Sexual offenders have lower rates of schizophrenia
    C. Sexual offenders have higher rates of psychotic disorders
    D. Only organic psychiatric conditions are more prevalent among sexual offenders
    E. Sexual offenders have a reduced risk of bipolar disorder

23. **Elderly offenders are often an under-researched population compared with working age offenders. Which of the following is true regarding elderly sex offenders?**
    A. Elderly sex offenders have higher rates of mental illness than non-sex offenders
    B. Elderly sex offenders have increased schizoid traits compared with non-sex offenders
    C. Sex offending in elderly people is associated more with organic brain disease
    D. Elderly sex offenders have increased antisocial traits compared with non-sex offenders
    E. There is an equal gender distribution among elderly sex offenders

24. **Which of the following statements is true with respect to reduction in the risk of violence associated with schizophrenia?**
    A. Newer antipsychotics reduce violence more than typical antipsychotics
    B. Violence risk is not modified by antipsychotic medications
    C. Medication adherence reduces risk of violence
    D. Olanzapine has the best evidence for reducing violence risk among atypical antipsychotics other than clozapine
    E. Typical antipsychotics increase the overall risk of violence

25. **The most important difference between legally determined non-insane automatisms and insane automatisms is**
    A. Treatability
    B. Recurrence risk
    C. Presence of intent
    D. Degree of crime
    E. Impulsivity

26. **With respect to morbid jealousy, the correct statement among the following is**
    A. It is always a delusional disorder
    B. It is coded separately in ICD-10
    C. It is coded separately in DSM-IV
    D. It is classified as a paraphilia
    E. It is associated with amphetamine use

27. The most common relationship a victim may have with his/her stalker is

A. Ex-partner
B. Employer
C. Medical practitioner
D. Unrelated stranger
E. Casual acquaintance

28. Which of the following ICD-10 diagnoses has a well-demonstrated causal association leading to stalking behaviour?

A. Obsessive–compulsive disorder
B. Delusional disorder
C. Depressive disorder
D. Organic brain disorders
E. Pervasive developmental disorder

29. It is found that criminal parents are at higher risk of having delinquent children. Which of the following is a correct statement in this regard?

A. Most criminal parents directly encourage crime in their children
B. Most criminal parents do not mind if their children commit a criminal offence
C. Findings of genetic transmission in delinquency have been shown to be robust
D. Poor parental supervision from criminal parents increases delinquency rates
E. Parents and children get convicted for the same crime more often than not

30. All of the following features are supportive of violence occurring during epileptic automatism except

A. Violent behaviour provoked by the victim
B. Presence of impaired consciousness
C. Poorly directed behaviour
D. Stereotyped motor acts preceding violent behaviour
E. Evidence of amnesia for the behaviour

31. An offender with a history of repeated arson admits to deliberate fire-setting, which is preceded by a certain degree of arousal. He has had a fascination with fire since childhood and achieves a sense of gratification when setting fires. He does not have antisocial personality disorder or substance use. The most appropriate diagnosis is

A. Obsessive compulsive disorder
B. Pyromania
C. Intellectual disability
D. Intermittent explosive disorder
E. Sadistic personality disorder

32. During the proceedings of a court trial it becomes evident that a murder victim had the habit of achieving sexual excitement from being humiliated and beaten after being bound and verbally abused. This is consistent with
    A. Voyeurism
    B. Sadism
    C. Masochism
    D. Fetishism
    E. Hypoxyphilia

33. In people with kleptomania which of the following medications has been demonstrated to be the most useful in double-blinded randomized controlled trials?
    A. Fluoxetine
    B. Olanzapine
    C. Lithium
    D. Naloxone
    E. None of the above

34. The proportion of adults with a history of childhood conduct disorder who satisfy the criteria for antisocial personality disorder in cross-sectional interviews is
    A. 75%
    B. 10%
    C. 20%
    D. 3%
    E. 95%

35. Among all homicides committed by those with psychotic illnesses, the proportion committed by those with a first episode psychosis and receiving no treatment is
    A. 1 in 10
    B. 2 in 10
    C. 4 in 10
    D. 7 in 10
    E. 9 in 10

36. Among various mental disorders seen in shoplifters, the strongest association is seen for
    A. Borderline personality disorder
    B. Antisocial personality disorder
    C. Schizophrenia
    D. Depression
    E. Kleptomania

37. **A 43-year-old patient with a diagnosis of delusional disorder reveals that he intends to 'rip off' his neighbour, with whom he believes that his wife is having an affair. Which of the following is correct with regard to management of this patient?**

    A. Police must not be informed to preserve confidentiality; wife can be informed
    B. Wife must not be informed to preserve confidentiality; police must be informed
    C. Police, wife, and, if needed, the neighbour must be informed
    D. Only the neighbour must be informed as there are no thoughts to harm the wife
    E. No one needs to be informed if the patient is legally detained in a hospital

38. **The proportion of prisoners in English prisons with one or other diagnosable mental disorder is**

    A. 30%
    B. 15%
    C. 45%
    D. 90%
    E. 5%

39. **All of the following are true with regard to suicide of a homicide perpetrator except**

    A. The suicide usually occurs within a week of murder
    B. It most commonly follows domestic homicides
    C. It follows child homicides more often than adult homicides
    D. It is most commonly associated with bipolar disorder
    E. An altruistic motive may be seen in elderly people

40. **In UK prisons, the most common method of committing suicide is**

    A. Hanging
    B. Poisoning
    C. Jumping from a height
    D. Gunshot injuries
    E. Self-immolation

41. **In which of the following settings are anatomical dolls used to aid interview?**

    A. Interviewing a learning-disabled adult for criminal offence
    B. Interviewing a child for diagnosing conduct disorder
    C. Interviewing an adult perpetrator of child abuse
    D. Interviewing a child for the possibility of sexual abuse
    E. Interviewing a child with suspected gender identity disorder

42. **A patient with chronic schizophrenia has improved core signs and symptoms. His remaining symptoms are of such low intensity that they no longer interfere significantly with his behaviour. The burden of current symptoms is such that if assessed now using standard criteria, he would not be diagnosed as having schizophrenia, although his social and vocational functioning has not altered much over the course of treatment. Which of the following correctly describes this state?**

   A. Recovery
   B. Remission
   C. Deficit state
   D. Lucid interval
   E. Recrudescence

43. **While measuring non-adherence to psychotropic medications, which of the following groups provides a subjective overestimate of the true adherence rates?**

   A. Patient group
   B. Doctors treating the patients
   C. Pharmacist
   D. Both A and B
   E. None of the above

44. **According to the European schizophrenia cohort study, homelessness experienced by patients with schizophrenia is highest in**

   A. Germany
   B. France
   C. Great Britain
   D. Belgium
   E. Turkey

45. **Which of the following is the major principle behind the original development of assertive community treatment?**

   A. Transfer of learnt social skills from the hospital to community setting is difficult
   B. Social skills training in the hospital setting is costly
   C. Training in community living is not a necessary component of rehabilitation
   D. Vocational rehabilitation can only take place in the community
   E. Cost of inpatient management is higher than the cost of community management

46. **Subjective measures of quality of life (QOL) in patients with mental illness may be inaccurate because of**

   A. QOL scales always include depression and anxiety items
   B. Reduced expectations may lead to claims of good QOL
   C. QOL is not measurable using questionnaires
   D. Subjective measures of QOL are not standardized
   E. Response rate for subjective QOL measures is very low

47. **Which of the following projects refers to promoting spontaneous recovery in schizophrenia without compulsory use of psychotropics?**

   A. Henderson hospital project
   B. Soteria project
   C. Partial hospitalization project
   D. Utopia project
   E. Melbourne PACE project

48. **According to the health belief model of treatment compliance, patients consider all of the following factors when deciding upon treatment adherence except**

   A. Susceptibility to illness
   B. Severity of illness
   C. Perceived benefits
   D. Probability of side-effects
   E. Social criticism

49. **The vocational rehabilitation programme with best evidence in schizophrenia is**

   A. Sheltered employment model
   B. Supported employment model
   C. Clubhouse model
   D. Skills training model
   E. Token economy model

50. **The proportion of patients of working age with serious mental health problems who are employed actively in the UK is**

   A. 10%
   B. 50%
   C. 40%
   D. 75%
   E. 1%

1. E.   Various types of studies have been hitherto employed to study the association between recorded crime and psychosis. One must remember that officially recorded crime may only be the tip of the proverbial iceberg in such studies. Various regional policies, jurisdictions, and practices affect the rate of recorded crime; in any case, these rates are not a true reflection of violence in the society. Many such studies have consistently found that a narrow diagnosis of schizophrenia or much broader psychosis have an increased risk of both non-violent and violent offending; this risk is greatest and most consistent for violent offences.

Murray R, et al., eds. *Essential Psychiatry*, 4th edn. Cambridge University Press, 2008, p. 541.

2. E.   The risk factors associated with violence in mental illness is a favourite topic in MRCPsych exams. It has been cogently shown that the magnitude of risk associated with a combination of factors such as male sex, young age, and lower socioeconomic status in a mentally 'well' person with no psychiatric history is higher than the risk of violence presented by mental disorders *per se*. Despite varied research, the causal pathway from mental illness to violence is still poorly sketched. The most consistently established risk factors that further increase the risk of violence among schizophrenia patients are (a) comorbid substance abuse, (b) comorbid personality disorder, (c) non-compliance with medication, and (d) active psychotic symptoms. Depression does not seem to be a major mediator of violence in schizophrenia patients.

Walsh E, Buchanan A and Fahy T. Violence and schizophrenia: examining the evidence. *British Journal of Psychiatry* 2002; **180**: 490–495.
Murray R, et al., eds. *Essential Psychiatry*, 4th edn. Cambridge University Press, 2008, p. 544.

3. E.   Most schizophrenia patients do not offend in direct response to delusions or hallucinations, although homicide offenders may be over-represented in those who are actively psychotic at the time of the offence. In general, schizophrenia patients who offend tend to have long histories of substance misuse, conduct problems, and delinquency, with extensive non-violent and violent offending prior to the onset of illness. Thus, the tendency to reoffend does not fall after a diagnosis of schizophrenia. The basic tenet one needs to remember regarding the epidemiology of violence in schizophrenia is that those risk factors for violence which operate in subjects without mental illness also operate in patients with schizophrenia.

Murray R, et al., eds. *Essential Psychiatry*, 4th edn. Cambridge University Press, 2008, p. 544.

4. B. Most research in forensic psychiatry has examined the relative risk of violence among the mentally ill compared with the general population. The population-attributable risk fraction (PAR%) refers to the percentage of violence in the population that can be ascribed to schizophrenia and thus could be eliminated if schizophrenia were eliminated from the population. Fazel and Grann (2006) reported that the population-attributable risk varied by gender and age in a given population. Overall, the PAR% of violence for psychiatric patients was 5.2%, suggesting that patients with severe mental illness commit 1 in 20 violent crimes. These data were obtained from analysing Swedish health registers between 1988 and 2000. This value may vary between countries and across various generations of birth cohorts.

Fazel S and Grann M. The population impact of severe mental illness on violent crime. *American Journal of Psychiatry* 2006; **163**: 1397–1403.

5. D. The population-attributable risk of violence in those with schizophrenia is a more important public health measure than relative risk as it indicates how much violence/crime could be eliminated if mental illness is 'eliminated'. It provides an easier and more accurate reflection than relative risk for the general public. When the crime rates in a society increase, the population-attributable risk due to any mental illness reduces. The population-attributable risk fraction of violence for mental illness rate is estimated as 5% using Swedish registers; this suggests that most crimes in Europe are not related to mental illness.

Murray R, *et al.*, eds. *Essential Psychiatry*, 4th edn. Cambridge University Press, 2008, p. 544.

6. D. The killing of a child by its mother is very rare and is called filicide. It is linked to depressive disorders more than any other mental illness. Patricide refers to the act of killing one's father. Sororicide is the act of killing one's sister. Matricide is the killing of one's mother and mariticide is killing of one's spouse. Fraternicide refers to killing one's brother.

Murray R, *et al.*, eds. *Essential Psychiatry*, 4th edn. Cambridge University Press, 2008, p. 545.

7. B. The five criteria currently used in court in England and Wales to determine fitness to plead have remained unchanged for over 150 years. These are collectively termed Pritchard's criteria: (1) ability to plead; (2) ability to understand evidence; (3) ability to understand the court proceedings; (4) ability to instruct a lawyer; (5) knowing that a juror can be challenged.

As the degree of mental illness can vary with time, its effect on fitness to stand trial can differ. Hence it is important to establish fitness/unfitness in the defendant as applicable at the time of the trial proceedings.

Rogers TP, Blackwood NJ, Farnham F., *et al*. Fitness to plead and competence to stand trial: a systematic review of the constructs and their application. *Journal of Forensic Psychiatry and Psychology* 2008; **19**: 576–596.

8. E. In the UK, the Bolam test has been the benchmark for assessing professional negligence since 1957. According to the Bolam test, 'A doctor is not guilty of negligence if he has acted in accordance with a practice accepted as proper by a responsible body of medical men skilled in that particular art'. In other words, a doctor is not negligent if he is acting in accordance with such a practice, merely because there is a body of opinion that takes a contrary view. McNaughton's test refers to the assessment of diminished responsibility in the wake of mental illness in court. The MacArthur competency assessment tool and Pritchard's criteria are used for assessing fitness to plead. Hare's checklist is used for the assessment of psychopathy.

Jones JW. The healthcare professional and the Bolam test. *British Dental Journal* 2000; **188**: 237–240.

9. B. If a defendant is found unfit to plead the likelihood of becoming fit is initially considered. If this is likely, e.g. following treatment, then the trial can be adjourned until such improvement occurs. If such improvement is unlikely, a jury trial of the facts takes place in the defendant's absence to determine whether the individual committed the alleged crime. If the individual is unfit to plead but at the end of the trial of facts it is established that he/she has committed the act, then one or other form of court disposal (e.g. a hospital order, supervision order or absolute discharge) is given.

Murray R, et al., eds. *Essential Psychiatry*, 4th edn. Cambridge University Press, 2008, p. 557.

10. D. HCR-20 (historical, clinical, risk management – 20) incorporates static historical risk factors, such as previous violence and early maladjustment, together with dynamic factors that may be particularly important in individual cases, such as level of insight and lack of personal support. It is a commonly used structured clinical risk assessment scale. VRAG is an actuarial tool that incorporates important predictors of reconviction studied in a sample of Canadian male offenders with mental disorder followed up for 7 years. PCL-R stands for the revised version of psychopathy checklist. It is used with HCR-20; it is not a stand-alone risk assessment instrument. MMPI is used as a psychometric tool for personality variables. The Iterative Classification Tree is an actuarial decision-making tool produced by Monahan et al. (2001) using data from the MacArthur risk assessment study. This tool uses many different combinations of bivariate risk factors to classify a person as high or low risk.

Dolan M and Doyle M. Violence risk prediction. Clinical and actuarial measures and the role of the Psychopathy Checklist. *British Journal of Psychiatry*, 2000; **177**: 303–311.

Monahan J. and Silver E. Judicial decision thresholds for violence risk management. *International Journal of Forensic Mental Health* 2003; **2**: 1–16.

11. C. VRAG is an actuarial risk tool that incorporates 12 items which are scored on the basis of a weighting procedure developed from the original study of Canadian prisoners. The variable with the heaviest weighting is the PCL-R psychopathy score, which is incorporated as a subscale. It does not use HCR-20 as a subscale. The factors positively associated with increased risk of recidivism are psychopathy score, history of elementary school difficulties, diagnosis of a personality disorder, young age, separation from parents prior to age 16, failure on prior conditional release, history of non-violent offences, never been married, and history of alcohol abuse. A diagnosis of schizophrenia is considered to reduce the overall risk of recidivism.

Dolan M and Doyle M. Violence risk prediction. Clinical and actuarial measures and the role of the Psychopathy Checklist. *British Journal of Psychiatry* 2000; **177**: 303–311.

12. E. Significantly below average intellectual ability is an independent predictor of future offending, irrespective of a diagnosis of learning disability (LD). Individuals with mild LD show a higher rate of offending than age- and sex-matched individuals without LD. No correlation has been found between the severity of intellectual disadvantage and the seriousness of the offence committed. In fact, individuals with more severe or profound learning disability rarely commit serious offences. Studies in the UK have shown a rate of 2–5% for recorded offences among the learning-disabled population. The degree of disability does not correlate with rate of offending. The most common offences by the learning-disabled group are property offences. Many risk factors that operate in the general population for risk of violence operate in the learning-disabled population, e.g. being young and male, a history of family offending, being unemployed, drug use, psychosocial disadvantage, etc.

Riding B, Swann C and Swann B, eds. *The Handbook of Forensic Learning Disabilities*. Radcliffe Publishing 2005, p. 124.

13. E.   Almost 80% of male remand prisoners in England and Wales were found to have at least one personality disorder, with antisocial personality disorder being most prevalent. From the Office of National Statistics data (1997) the prevalence of any personality disorder was 78% for male remand prisoners, 64% for male sentenced prisoners and 50% for female prisoners (both sentenced and remand).

Antisocial personality disorder had the highest prevalence of any category of personality disorder (63% of male remand prisoners, 49% of male sentenced prisoners, and 31% of female prisoners) followed by paranoid personality disorder in men (29% of male remand prisoners, 20% of male sentenced, and 16% of female prisoners) and borderline personality disorder in women (20% of female prisoners). Compare these rates with a weighted prevalence for any personality disorder of 4.4% among people aged 16–74 years in households in England, Scotland and Wales.

Coid J, Yang M, Tyrer P et al. Prevalence and correlates of personality disorder in Great Britain. *The British Journal of Psychiatry* 2006; **188**: 423–431.

Singleton N, Meltzer, H., Gatward, R, et al. *Psychiatric Morbidity among Prisoners in England and Wales*. Stationery Office, 1998.

14. D.   The McNaughton rules refer to a set of guidelines for the insanity defence that was used in England until the 1960s. According to these rules one can plead the defence of insanity only if 'at the time of committing the act, the accused was labouring under such a defect of reason from disease of the mind, as not to know the nature and quality of the act he was doing, or if he did know it then he did not know he was doing what was wrong'. Those who merely lack the capacity to control a criminal action could still be deemed punishable. Hence, a defect of moral judgement or failure to exercise existing capability to make the right decision cannot be brought up as an insanity defence under the McNaughton rules.

Murray R, Kendler K, et al., eds. *Essential Psychiatry*, 4th edn. Cambridge University Press, 2008, p. 558.

15. E.   The constructs of psychopathy and antisocial or dissocial personality are often referred to interchangeably, but in reality these are quite different concepts. Approximately 3–5% of people in the general population would meet the criteria for antisocial personality. But less than 1% will meet the criteria for psychopathy (i.e. a high score (30/40) on the PCL-R). Similarly, although only 15% of male prisoners have scores that fall in the psychopathy range on the PCL-R, nearly 80% of them will satisfy the criteria for antisocial personality disorder. In other words, although most patients (81%) diagnosed as psychopaths by the PCL-R criteria met the criteria for a diagnosis of antisocial personality disorder, only a minority (nearly 35–40%) of those with antisocial personality receive a diagnosis of PCL-R psychopathy. The correlation between antisocial personality disorder and PCL-R scores was much higher for behavioural (social deviance: $r = 0.65$) factor of psychopathy than affective (interpersonal: $r = 0.39$) factor. Psychopaths are less impulsively aggressive than those with antisocial personality disorder, but are more likely to engage in antisocial behaviour of an instrumental nature. Those with psychopathy commit higher rates of serious violence and have strikingly high rates of recidivism than those with antisocial personality disorder but who are not psychopathic.

Ogloff JRP. Psychopathy/antisocial personality disorder conundrum. *Australian and New Zealand Journal of Psychiatry* 2006; **40**: 519–528.

Murray R, Kendler K et al., eds. *Essential Psychiatry*, 4th edn. Cambridge University Press, 2008, p. 547.

16. A. Various neurobiological findings have been demonstrated in those with psychopathy. These include impairments in appreciation of the emotional significance of external experience, strikingly low levels of baseline and reactive autonomic arousal and reduced fear-based learning. Although impaired verbal abilities have been demonstrated as a consistent risk factor for serious antisocial and delinquent behaviour, those with psychopathic traits often show serious antisocial behaviour, despite showing no impairment in their verbal abilities. In fact, Individuals who were high on callous–unemotional traits (a feature of psychopathy) with higher scores on the measure of verbal abilities reported the greatest violent delinquency in a sample of adolescent delinquents. For non-psychopathic individuals, a significant difference in P300 amplitude was noted between target and non-target stimuli. But in psychopathic individuals reliable P300 amplitude differences between the target and non-target visual conditions were not seen.

Muñoz LC, Frick PJ, Kimonis ER, *et al.* Verbal ability and delinquency: testing the moderating role of psychopathic traits. *Journal of Child Psychology and Psychiatry* 2008; **49**: 414–421.
Kiehl KA, Hare RD, Liddle PF, McDonald JJ. Reduced P300 responses in criminal psychopaths during a visual oddball task. *Biological Psychiatry* 1999; **45**: 1498–1507.

17. E. Even in those who are violent but do not have a demonstrable mental illness, the likelihood of having had a neurodevelopmental insult is high. This is shown by the presence of higher rates of minor physical anomalies in violently delinquent adolescents. Similarly, higher rates of neurological soft signs, maternal smoking during pregnancy, and obstetric complications have also been demonstrated. Defects in executive functioning and impulse control have also been shown to correlate with violence in the non-mentally ill samples.

Murray R, Kendler K *et al.*, eds. *Essential Psychiatry*, 4th edn. Cambridge University Press, 2008, p. 549.

18. B. Children differ in their response to maltreatment in terms of future risk of criminal behaviour. Although maltreatment increases the risk of later criminality by about 50%, most maltreated children do not become delinquents or adult criminals. It is possible that certain genetic susceptibility factors could influence the causal pathway. Caspi *et al.* demonstrated that the effect of childhood maltreatment on antisocial behaviour was significantly weaker among males with high *MAO-A* activity than among males with low *MAO-A* activity. It was also shown that girls with a low *MAO-A* activity genotype but not those with high *MAO-A* activity were more likely to develop conduct disorder if they were maltreated. Hence, high *MAO-A* activity has a protective influence against maltreatment for both sexes.

Caspi A, McClay J, Moffitt TE, *et al.* Role of genotype in the cycle of violence in maltreated children. *Science* 2002; **297**: 851–854.

19. A. Depending on the definitions used, the rates of 'mental disorder' vary greatly among homicide offenders. The national confidential inquiry into suicide and homicide by people with mental illness in the UK established the frequency of mental illness in a complete national sample of homicides as 44% (lifetime history of mental disorder). At the time of the homicide, 14% had symptoms of mental illness. The most frequent diagnosis was personality disorder (11%), closely followed by alcohol dependence (10%) and drug dependence. Among major mental illnesses, affective disorders (10%) were more common than schizophrenia (7%).

Shaw J, Hunt IM, Flynn S, *et al.* Rates of mental disorder in people convicted of homicide. National clinical survey. *British Journal of Psychiatry* 2006; **188**: 143–147.

20. B.   From the national confidential inquiry on homicide (1996–9) data, only 8–11% of the total sample of all homicide offenders (n=1594) were in contact with mental health services at some time in the preceding year. The main diagnoses in those with any previous contact with mental health services were schizophrenia (24%), personality disorder (18%), and depressive disorder (16%). Psychiatric reports were not available for nearly one-quarter of all homicide cases.

Shaw J, Hunt IM, Flynn S, *et al.* Rates of mental disorder in people convicted of homicide. National clinical survey. *British Journal of Psychiatry* 2006; **188**: 143–147.

21. E.   The national confidential inquiry on homicide (1996–9) data found that 22% of all reported homicides were stranger homicides. In stranger homicides the perpetrator was more likely to be a young male and less likely to have a history of mental disorder or a history of contact with mental health services. They were also less likely to have psychiatric symptoms at the time of the offence than perpetrators of non-stranger homicides. They were more likely to have a history of drug or alcohol misuse.

Shaw J, Amos T, Hunt IM, *et al.* Mental illness in people who kill strangers: longitudinal study and national clinical survey. *British Medical Journal* 2004; **328**: 734–737.

22. C.   Traditional expert views on the association between sexual offending and psychiatric disorders were challenged by a case–control study using 13 years' data from Swedish crime registers conducted by Fazel *et al* (2007). The authors compared sexual offenders with a random sample of men from the general population and reported that sexual offenders were more likely to have been hospitalized for a psychiatric condition than men in the general population (odds ratio (OR) 6.3). They also showed that sexual offenders were more likely to have a severe mental illness, including schizophrenia (OR 4.8), bipolar disorder (OR 3.4), other psychoses (OR 5.2), or an organic psychiatric condition (OR 2.4).

Fazel S, Sjostedt G, Langstrom N, *et al.* Severe mental illness and risk of sexual offending in men: a case-control study based on Swedish national registers. *Jornal of Clinical Psychiatry* 2007; **68**: 588–596.

23. B.   As stated in the question, research is scarce in the area of criminality in elderly people. A case–control study comparing elderly sex offenders with elderly non-sex offenders showed that the rates of psychotic illness, depressive disorders, personality disorders, and dementia did not differ significantly between the two groups. Significant differences were observed at the level of personality traits wherein sex offenders were observed to have more schizoid, obsessive–compulsive, and avoidant traits but fewer antisocial traits than non-sex offenders. Similar to any other age group of sex offenders, the elderly group consisted exclusively of males. The authors concluded that sex offending in elderly people is associated more with personality factors than with mental illness or organic brain disease.

Fazel S, Hope T, O'Donnell I and Jacoby R. Psychiatric, demographic and personality characteristics of elderly sex offenders. *Psychological Medicine* 2002; **32**: 219–226.

24. C.   The data from Clinical Antipsychotic Trials of Intervention Effectiveness (CATIE) project were analysed for the effect of antipsychotics on violent behaviour in those with schizophrenia. Violence declined from 16% to 9% in those who completed the antipsychotic treatment throughout the trial period of 6 months. But no demonstrable difference was found among the different medication groups; medication adherence was associated with a reduced risk of violence only in patients with no history of childhood antisocial conduct. Hence the effect of antipsychotics on violence in schizophrenia seems to depend on the effect of the drugs on acute psychopathology. This study did not show an advantage for second-generation antipsychotics in violence risk reduction when compared with first-generation antipsychotic perphenazine.

Swanson JW, Swartz MS, Van Dorn RA, *et al*. Comparison of antipsychotic medication effects on reducing violence in people with schizophrenia. *British Journal of Psychiatry* 2008; **193**: 37–43.

25. B.   Automatism is a psychiatric defence used in cases of homicide. Under automatism, the defence counsel argues that the accused person's behaviour at the time of the offence was 'automatic'. In other words, *mens rea* was absent and the act was merely done without the conscious force of the mind – no intention was present. Some causes of automatism include hypoglycaemia, sleep walking, epilepsy, etc. In general, the defendant is acquitted if he/she is found to have a case of sane automatism, i.e. automatisms that occur due to external causes; these are unlikely to recur, hence the acquittal. Insane automatisms are due to 'internal diseases' or disorders of the mind, which have a propensity to recur. This classification is purely legal and not based on the impulsive nature of the crime or treatability of the condition. Note that both types of automatisms, by definition, mean that there is a lack of intent (*mens rea*). Often discrete medical disorders can be classified in either type of automatism.

Murray R, Kendler K, *et al*., eds. *Essential Psychiatry*, 4th edn. Cambridge University Press, 2008, p. 558.

26. E.   Morbid jealousy (also known as Othello syndrome) may be a presenting feature of schizophrenia, delusional disorder, organic brain syndromes, or affective psychosis. It is not coded separately in ICD-10 or DSM-IV but as a subtype of delusional disorder; the delusion of infidelity is described by both systems of classification. Alcohol, amphetamine, or cocaine use can give rise to delusions of jealousy that may develop into full-blown delusional disorder in vulnerable individuals.

Kingham M, Gordon H. Aspects of morbid jealousy. *Advances in Psychiatric Treatment* 2004; **10**: 207–215.

27. A.   Using a broad definition of stalking the British Crime Survey (2000) estimated that 2.9% of adults aged 16–59 had been stalked in the preceding year. Women (4.0%) were more likely to be victims of stalking/harassment than men (1.7%). Risks were particularly high for young women aged between 16 and 19 (16.8%). About a third of incidents were perpetrated by someone who was in an intimate relationship with the victim at the start of the episode or in the past. A community-based epidemiological study on stalking from a medium-sized German city reported that most of the stalking victims (32%) were pursued by former intimate partners.

Budd T, Mattinson J. The extent and nature of stalking: findings from the 1998 British Crime Survey. Home Office; 2000.
Dressing H, Kuehner C, Gass P. Lifetime prevalence and impact of stalking in a European population. *British Journal of Psychiatry* 2005; **187**: 168–172.

28. B. Delusional disorder or erotomanic type has a well-known link with stalking behaviour. An often-cited descriptive study of stalking was carried out by Mullen *et al.* (1999) in a group of 145 stalkers referred to a psychiatric centre. Mullen grouped stalkers into rejected, intimacy-seeking, incompetent, resentful, and predatory types. These are arbitrary and not entirely exclusive groupings, although such typology helps in predicting the likely nature and duration of stalking and the risk of assault to a certain extent. Among these, the rejected stalkers make up the largest group, formed predominantly of ex-partners. The predatory stalkers form a small group with a high potential for sexual violence. Mullen described incompetent stalkers as 'intellectually limited and socially incompetent individuals with rudimentary courting rituals' whose victims do not reciprocate their affection. Resentful stalkers tend to frighten and distress the victim because of a sense of grievance. The intimacy-seeking stalkers form a spectrum, from those with erotomania to those with rigid infatuations. The erotomanic delusions could be both secondary to pre-existing psychotic disorders such as schizophrenia and as part of a delusional disorder.

Mullen PE, Pathé M, Purcell R, Stuart GW. Study of stalkers. *American Journal of Psychiatry* 1999; **156**: 1244–1249.

29. D. It is well established that having a convicted mother, father, brother, or sister significantly predicts juvenile delinquency in boys. Thus intergenerational continuity in offending has been noted. There is no evidence that criminal parents directly encourage their children to commit crime; in fact, most convicted men disagreed with the statement that 'I would not mind if my son/daughter committed a criminal offence'. Epidemiological studies have shown that it was extremely rare for a parent and a child to be convicted for an offence committed together. Thus, the major mediator between parental criminality and juvenile delinquency seems to be poor parental supervision, with some role for genetic transmission of antisocial behaviour.

Farrington, D.P. (1995). The development of offending and antisocial behaviour from childhood: key findings from the Cambridge Study in Delinquent Development. *Journal of Child Psychology and Psychiatry*, 36, 929–64.

30. A. Violent acts during epilepsy are extremely uncommon. But epileptic automatisms have been invoked as a defence in courts time and again. Most cases involved spontaneous, non-directed, stereotyped aggressive movements, with violence against property being more common than inflicting serious bodily injuries. Severe violence, if seen at all, is largely restricted to postictal states. When aggression presents as a feature of an epileptic seizure, it usually begins suddenly without provocation, lasts only for brief periods, and ends abruptly with evidence of impaired consciousness during the act. The act usually does not involve detailed or interactive behaviour but appears stereotyped. Episodes of postictal or ictal violence are usually associated with amnesia for the event.

Marsh L, Krauss GL. Aggression and violence in patients with epilepsy. *Epilepsy and Behavior* 2000; **1**: 160–168.

31. B. Pyromania is an extremely rare disorder that presents with repeated fire-setting. It is recognized as a category in both ICD-10 and DSM-IV, under impulse control disorders. The diagnostic criteria include tension or affective arousal before the act of setting the fire, fascination with, interest in, curiosity about, or attraction to fire and its situational contexts, as well as pleasure, gratification, or relief when setting fires or when witnessing or participating in the aftermath of a fire.

Lindberg N, Holi M, Tani P, Virkkunen M. Looking for pyromania: characteristics of a consecutive sample of Finnish male criminals with histories of recidivist fire-setting between 1973 and 1993. *BMC Psychiatry* 2005; **5**: 47.

32. C.   Masochism refers to a paraphilia characterized by persistent interest in sexual activities that demean, humiliate, or cause suffering to self. Masochism requires a partner who complies by dominating and inflicting suffering. In contrast, sadism refers to a paraphilia wherein sexual arousal and gratification are obtained by inflicting pain and suffering upon the partner. Hence a sadist and a masochist can be mutual partners. Voyeurism is characterized by achieving gratification by watching people undressing or having sexual intercourse. It is the most common paraphilia reported. Fetishism refers to compulsive sexual interest in inanimate objects that are often worn by or associated with sexual partners. Hypoxyphilia (autoerotic asphyxiation) is not separately coded as a paraphilia in ICD/DSM; it refers to a specific form of masochism in which sexual arousal is attained by self-suffocation, e.g. via hanging while masturbating.

Millon T, Blaney PH, Davis RD, eds. *Oxford Textbook of Psychopathology*. Oxford University Press, 1999, p. 422.

33. E.   Kleptomania is considered by some as part of the obsessive–compulsive spectrum. Extending the effectiveness of selective serotonin reuptake inhibitors (SSRI) in obsessive compulsive spectrum disorders, several case series of successful SSRI use in kleptomania have appeared. A response rate of nearly 80% at week 7 was reported for kleptomania in an open-label trial of escitalopram; this was not maintained to the same degree in a subsequent double-blind placebo-controlled discontinuation trial. Naltrexone and mood stabilizers have also been studied in open-label trials for kleptomania, with variable benefits. To date, no strong evidence from randomized controlled trials exists to support pharmacological interventions in kleptomania.

Koran LM, Aboujaoude EN, Gamel NN. Escitalopram treatment of kleptomania: an open-label trial followed by double-blind discontinuation. *Journal of Clinical Psychiatry* 2007; **68**: 422–427.

34. A.   Traditionally it was thought that 40% of those with conduct disorder experience lifetime persistence of traits that are termed as antisocial personality disorder. But this has been now challenged to be an underestimate; data from the National Epidemiologic Survey on Alcohol and Related Conditions (NESARC) in the USA suggests that nearly 75% of adults who were retrospectively identified to have had conduct disorder as children satisfied current criteria for antisocial personality disorder. Although this is a retrospective design, the estimates are from a more representative sample than older retrospective studies.

Gelhorn HL, Sakai JT, Price RK, Crowley TJ. DSM-IV conduct disorder criteria as predictors of antisocial personality disorder. *Comprehensive Psychiatry* 2007; **48**: 529–538.

35. C.   The prevalence of schizophrenic disorders in the general population is below 1%, but patients with schizophrenia constitute between 5% and 20% of all homicide offenders. An increased risk of homicide has been associated with the first episode of psychosis. A meta-analysis of studies reporting homicide offences in psychotic patients showed that 38.5% of homicides occurred during the first episode of psychosis, prior to initial treatment. The rate ratio of homicide in the first episode of psychosis was 15.5 times the annual rate of homicide after treatment for psychosis. Nearly 40% of patients with schizophrenia who commit homicides do not have any history of psychiatric care.

Nielssen O, Large M. Rates of homicide during the first episode of psychosis and after treatment: a systematic review and meta-analysis. Schizophrenia Bulletin 2008; doi:10.1093/schbul/sbn144.

36. B. Shoplifting is different from kleptomania: the former is a broadly defined behaviour whereas the latter is a specific psychiatric diagnostic category. Data from a national study carried out in the USA (National Epidemiologic Survey on Alcohol and Related Conditions) have demonstrated that most individuals (nearly 90%) who admitted to at least one episode of lifetime shoplifting had a lifetime history of at least one psychiatric diagnosis, compared with nearly 50% in non-shoplifters. In both groups, the most prevalent disorders were nicotine dependence and alcohol use disorders, with nearly three or four times increased risk respectively; among shoplifters, the strongest associations were found for antisocial personality disorder and substance use disorders. Kleptomania is a rare condition and occurs in less than 5% of identified shoplifters and less than 0.6% of the general population.

Blanco C, Grant J, Petry NM, *et al.* Prevalence and correlates of shoplifting in the united states: results from the national epidemiologic survey on alcohol and related conditions (NESARC). *American Journal of Psychiatry* 2008; **165**: 905–913.

37. C. In *Tarasoff* v *The Regents of the University of California et al.*, a case was brought by the parents of Tatiana Tarasoff, who had been murdered by Prosenjit Poddar. Poddar had previously disclosed his violent feelings against Tarasoff to Dr Moore, the campus psychologist. Although Dr Moore notified the police of his concerns about Poddar, the police released him after questioning. Ms Tarasoff and her family were not warned of the danger she faced. The court ruled that the clinician had a duty to protect and warn a third party from risk of harm from his/her patient, even though that third party was not under the clinician's clinical care. In the UK, a Tarasoff ruling does not apply directly; breach of confidentiality for the sake of public interest has been recognized. According to Tarasoff principles, the police and third parties must be warned of the risk as well as the wife.

Gavaghan C. A Tarasoff for Europe? A European Human Rights perspective on the duty to protect. *International Journal of Law and Psychiatry* 2007; **30**: 255–267.

38. D. Data from *Psychiatric Morbidity among Prisoners in England and Wales* 1998 showed that a large proportion of all prisoners had several mental disorders. Only 1 in 10 or fewer showed no evidence of any of the five disorders considered in the survey (personality disorder, psychosis, neurosis, alcohol misuse, and drug dependence). Thus the rate of psychiatric diagnosis was nearly 90% in prisons. Most prisoners who had a psychiatric diagnosis had more than one diagnosable condition; this was especially true if the primary diagnosis was psychotic illness. Rates for multiple disorders were higher among remand than sentenced prisoners. Despite this, most prisoners receive poor, if any, psychiatric services in prison.

Singleton N, Meltzer H, Gatward R, *et al* Psychiatric Morbidity among Prisoners in England and Wales. Stationery Office, 1998.

39. D. Homicide–suicides are mostly family affairs, especially when the perpetrator is female. Barraclough and Harris (2002) studied all murder–suicides over a 4-year period in the UK and found that 3% of male, 11% of female, and 19% of child homicides were of this type. Similarly, of all suicides, 0.8% male and 0.4% female deaths occurred as homicide–suicides. The typical cases involved families of low socioeconomic status. Death or fatal injury occurred on the same day in nearly 90% of incidents; in atypical cases the maximum interval between suicide and homicide was 10 months. In elderly people such homicide–suicide combinations are often suicide pacts complicated by depression or dementia in a couple or one of the partners. They can be considered altruistic, as often elderly people believe that the world will be better off without them.

Barraclough B, Harris EC. Suicide preceded by murder: the epidemiology of homicide. *Psychological Medicine* 2002; **32**: 577–584.

40. A. A 2-year national survey of prison suicides described the clinical and social circumstances of self-inflicted deaths among prisoners in England and Wales. Nearly one-third occurred within 7 days of arrival in prison. The commonest method (nearly 92%) was hanging or self-strangulation; nearly three-quarters had a history of mental disorder. The commonest primary diagnosis was drug dependence.

Shaw J, Baker D, Hunt IM, Moloney A, Appleby L. Suicide by prisoners: National clinical survey. *The British Journal of Psychiatry* 2004; **184**: 263–267.

41. D. Anatomical dolls are used in forensic investigation of children who are alleged victims of sexual abuse. Various procedures such as drawings, puppets, observation for sexualized behaviour, etc., have been used to obtain a child's report of sexual abuse. But research has not confirmed that responses supposedly indicative of abuse (e.g. drawing genitalia in human figure drawings, demonstrating intercourse, or oral sex between anatomical dolls, etc.) consistently occur with high frequency among abused children. Hence the use of such methods is controversial.

Dammeyer MD. The assessment of child sexual abuse allegations: using research to guide clinical decision making. *Behavioral Sciences and the Law.* 1998; **16**: 21–34.

42. B. The Remission in Schizophrenia Working Group defined remission 'as a state in which patients have experienced improvements in core signs and symptoms to the extent that any remaining symptoms are of such low intensity that they no longer interfere significantly with behaviour and are below the threshold typically utilized in justifying an initial diagnosis of schizophrenia'. Thus 'remission' is not the same as 'recovery', which is the ability to function in the community, socially and vocationally, as well as being relatively free of psychopathology. Accordingly, remission is a necessary but not sufficient step towards recovery. Note that such a scientific definition of recovery views recovery as a state of outcome; this is very different from the concept of recovery promulgated by consumer groups.

Bellack AS. Scientific and consumer models of recovery in schizophrenia: concordance, contrasts, and implications. *Schizophria Bulletin* 2006; **32**: 432–442.

43. D. In clinical practice, medication adherence is either assumed *de facto* or assessed from patients' self-reports. Both these measures of adherence have limited validity. Medication levels in body fluids are susceptible to manipulation. The use of electronic monitoring and a third party such as a pharmacist/clinical assistant to assess adherence may be more useful. Using the measurement of adherence as a dichotomous variable, a study comparing adherence estimates by patients, clinicians, and research assistants using electronic monitors was carried out. Compared with electronic monitoring, prescribers dramatically overestimated adherence levels. Electronic monitoring detected greater non-adherence rates (57%) than either prescribers (7%) or patients (5%), although independent third-party ratings were closer to electronic ratings (54%).

Byerly MJ, Thompson A, Carmody T, *et al.* Validity of electronically monitored medication adherence and conventional adherence measures in schizophrenia. *Psychiatric Services* 2007; **58**: 844–847.

44. C. Homelessness has a recognized association with severe mental illness. 'Rooflessness' refers to those living on the streets; it is difficult to include them in research surveys. Hence most researchers use a looser definition of having no fixed address and include people living in hostels and emergency accommodation. A broader term of 'housing instability' refers to the tenuousness of housing tenure. In the USA, community studies show that about a fifth of those with schizophrenia had no fixed address – a rate that was 2.4 times higher than for major depression. The European Schizophrenia Cohort (Bebbington *et al.*, 2005) found that 32.8% of the British sample had experienced homelessness in their lifetime compared with 8.4% in Germany and 12.9% in France. The rate in London was even higher (43%).

Kooyman I, Dean K, Harvey S, Walsh E. Outcomes of public concern in schizophrenia. *The British Journal of Psychiatry* 2007; **191**: s29–36.

Bebbington P, Angermeyer M, Azorin J-M, *et al.* The European Schizophrenia Cohort. *Social Psychiatry and Psychiatric Epidemiology* 2005; **40**: 707–717.

45. A. Assertive community treatment (ACT) was initially developed from the 'training in community living' programme at the Mendota Mental Health Institute in Madison, Wisconsin, by Marx, Stein, and Test. According to them community rehabilitation existent in the 1970s served only to maintain patients in 'a tenuous community adjustment on the brink of rehospitalization', instead of helping patients to meet all their needs. The key principle was to provide treatment in community settings, because skills learnt in the community can be better applied in the community. In the UK it has been shown that community mental health teams are able to support people with serious mental illnesses as effectively as ACT teams, but ACT may be better at engaging clients and may lead to greater satisfaction with services (UK-700 and REACT studies; see Burns *et al.* for more information). A systematic review of the evidence on the ACT model has suggested that the degree of reliance on hospitalization may be the key factor in heterogeneity of outcomes seen in ACT services: the higher the reliance on hospitalization in a community, the more effective the ACT-based services are for that community. Other options in the question are false. The cost of skills training is not a major factor behind the advocacy of the ACT model.

Burns T, Catty J, Dash M, *et al.* Use of intensive case management to reduce time in hospital in people with severe mental illness: systematic review and meta-regression. *British Medical Journal* 2007; **335**: 336–342.

46. B. QOL is measurable using questionnaires; these measures can be subjective or objective and many standardized instruments for both are available. Most but not all QOL instruments contain 'emotional' items, mostly relating to depression and anxiety. Such scales when applied to psychiatric conditions become tautological as the content of both measures largely overlap, e.g. the Quality of Life in Depression Scale (QLDS), which is made up mainly of depressive symptoms. Subjective measures of QOL in psychiatry are particularly problematic because of 'affective, cognitive or reality distortion fallacies'. A depressed patient may underestimate his true QOL; similarly, psychopathological states may lead to distorted appraisal of one's QOL. Hence external (e.g. relatives/carers) appraisal may be necessary to complement subjective QOLs in psychiatry. Another specific type of bias noted in QOL studies in psychiatry is what is termed as 'standard drift fallacy'. Quality of life can be thought of as the gap between a person's expectations and achievements. This gap can be kept minimal (i.e. good QOL) either by living up to one's expectations or lowering these expectations. Many patients with long-term mental disorders report being 'satisfied with life' in conditions that would be regarded as inadequate or unbearable by other factions of the society. This is due to the tendency of chronic mentally ill people to lower their standards over time and thus keep the gap between expectations and achievements narrow (falsely inflated subjective QOL).

Katschnig H. Quality of life in mental disorders: challenges for research and clinical practice. *World Psychiatry* 2006; **5**: 139–145.

47. B. Different models of therapeutic communities have been tried as alternatives to hospitalization for people diagnosed with schizophrenia. Some of these models emphasized the need for individuals to experience psychosis with minimal interference and high levels of support instead of early intervention with antipsychotic medication. In the UK, initiatives such as Kingsley Hall, associated with Laing, and Villa 21, associated with David Cooper, are examples. In the USA, the 'Soteria paradigm,' was developed by Mosher and colleagues; the critical elements of Soteria are provision of a small, community-based therapeutic milieu; significant lay person staffing; preservation of personal power and social networks; sustained communal responsibilities; a 'phenomenological' relational style (giving meaning to the subjective experience of psychosis by 'being with' and 'doing with' the client); and no or low-dose antipsychotic medication administered from a position of choice and without coercion. Henderson hospital is a therapeutic community for personality disorders, not schizophrenia. The PACE (Personal Assessment and Crisis Evaluation) Clinic is a centre for people with suspected incipient psychosis in Australia where trialled interventions aimed at preventing or delaying the onset of psychotic disorders are used; these interventions include psychological and social interventions, either alone or in combination with pharmacotherapy. Partial hospitalisation refers to mentalization-based therapy for borderline personality disorder.

Calton T, Ferriter M, Huband N, Spandler H. A Systematic review of the soteria paradigm for the treatment of people diagnosed with schizophrenia. *Schizophrenia Bulletin* 2008; **34**:181–192.

Yung AR, McGorry PD, Francey SM, *et al*. PACE: a specialised service for young people at risk of psychotic disorders. *Medical Journal of Australia* 2007; **187**: s43–46.

48. E. According to the health belief model four main belief categories have an impact on patients' compliance with prescribed treatment. These are (1) perceived benefits, (2) perceived costs, (3) perceived susceptibility to illness and cure, (4) secondary benefits of medication and adherence. This model emphasizes the patient's decision-making process, which is composed of a subjective cost–benefit analysis in the context of the patient's personal goals and priorities. Thus any changes in levels of adherence are possible only via alteration of the patient's perceptions. The more severe the illness, the higher the likelihood of perceived benefits. Social criticism does not constitute a major factor in adherence according to the health benefits model, unless avoiding it is perceived directly as a benefit by the patient.

Patel MX, David AS. Medication adherence: predictive factors and enhancement strategies. *Psychiatry* 2004; **3**: 41–44.

49. B.   Competitive employment rates are low in schizophrenia. People with mental health disorders represent the largest group (40%) who claim incapacity benefit. Various vocational programmes have been tried and tested in schizophrenia rehabilitation. Work acts as both a process and the outcome for rehabilitation in chronic schizophrenia. Sheltered employment refers to the traditional 'train and place model' where gradual stepwise skills training is initially carried out; when an individual makes sufficient progress, later placement is offered, often in sheltered workshops but not in competitive job markets. This approach remains the most widespread in Europe. Models that emphasize relatively quick placement in competitive jobs with continued support from employment specialists (supported employment models) are shown to have considerable impact compared with schemes that concentrate on social skills training or voluntary non-competitive work. This is the individual placement and support model in contrast to traditional stepwise support-till-placement (train and place approach) models. A multicentred RCT of Individual placement and training model (IPS) was carried out across six centres in Europe, including London. The results indicated that IPS was more effective than usual rehabilitation and vocational services for every work-related outcome, with 55% of patients assigned to IPS working for at least 1 day compared with 28% patients assigned to vocational services; the drop-out and readmission rates were comparatively lower in the IPS group. Local unemployment rates across the six centres accounted for a substantial amount of the heterogeneity in IPS effectiveness. Clubhouses offer an opportunity for a person with schizophrenia to resume an independent lifestyle with decent housing, facilities for education, job training, and placement via membership at a common daycentre. Token economy cannot be considered as a vocational model; it is a behavioural technique using secondary reinforcers (tokens) in rehabilitation units to enable desirable behaviour.

Burns T, Catty J, Becker T, et al. The effectiveness of supported employment for people with severe mental illness: a randomised controlled trial. *Lancet* 2007; **370**: 1146–1152.

50. A.   Annual (now quarterly) labour force surveys in the UK yield the rates of employment for the mentally ill population. Patients with a significant mental illness are among the most excluded in society. It is estimated that, at best, 15% of working age people with long-term mental health problems are working, far lower than any other group of disabled people. Even when working they work fewer hours and earn only two-thirds of the national average hourly rate. The employment rates for those with less serious mental health problems are relatively better at 20–25% but still people with mental disorders constitute 39% of all claimants of Disability Allowance and 34% of Incapacity Benefit, according to Department of Works and Pensions, UK. Joblessness and lack of social networks are often exacerbated by discrimination and profound loss of social status suffered by the mentally ill. Recovery from mental illness is significantly impeded by the above.

Huxley P, Thornicroft G. Social inclusion, social quality and mental illness. *British Journal of Psychiatry* 2003; **182**: 289–290.

1. **All of the following are features of Down's syndrome except**

   A. Increased cardiac mortality and morbidity
   B. Lax ligaments
   C. Wide gap between first and second toes
   D. Increased incidence of leukaemia
   E. Delayed puberty

2. **Which of the following is false with regard to behavioural and psychiatric disorders associated with Down's syndrome?**

   A. Rates of non-organic psychiatric disorders are higher in Down's syndrome than in learning disability due to other causes
   B. Autism has a significant association with Down's syndrome
   C. Seizures are a frequent clinical feature of Alzheimer's dementia in those with Down's syndrome
   D. Medical conditions may underlie psychiatric presentations
   E. Most patients have a placid temperament

3. **Classification of mental retardation into 'subcultural' and 'pathological' subtypes was first described by**

   A. EO Lewis
   B. Henry Maudsley
   C. Kraepelin
   D. Morel
   E. Kanner

4. **All of the following are true with regard to foetal alcohol syndrome except**

   A. Decreased cranial size at birth
   B. Agenesis of the corpus callosum
   C. Neurosensory hearing loss
   D. Poor eye–hand coordination
   E. Congenital cataract

5. **A subcultural rather than neuropathological explanation for learning disability is supported by which of the following?**

    A. Even distribution of learning disability across different socioeconomic groups of the population
    B. Existence of a profound degree of learning disability
    C. Learning disability in other members of the family
    D. Facial dysmorphic features
    E. Significant problems with adaptive functioning

6. **A 6-year-old boy has autistic features, hyperactivity, and inattention. He is noted to have frequent self-injurious head banging and nail pulling. There is a history of both nocturnal and diurnal enuresis. He has an IQ in the range of moderate learning disability. He has normal uric acid levels in his serum. The most likely cause is**

    A. Trisomy 21
    B. 7q11 deletion in the elastin gene
    C. 17p11 microdeletion
    D. Hypoxanthine guanine phosphoribosyltransferase deficiency
    E. Trisomy 13

7. **The most powerful predictor of overall functional outcome in children with autism is given by**

    A. Family history of autism
    B. Autistic symptom count
    C. Presence of soft neurological signs
    D. IQ level
    E. Non-verbal skills

8. **Which of the following groups of school children develops a higher prevalence of psychopathology as adults than the others listed?**

    A. Victims of bullying
    B. Perpetrators of bullying
    C. Children who do not bully and are not victimized by others
    D. Children who frequently bully others and get victimized by others
    E. Children who report bullying to teachers and authorities

9. **The most common known inherited cause of learning disability is**

    A. Down's syndrome
    B. Fragile X syndrome
    C. Cri du chat syndrome
    D. Galactosaemia
    E. Hypothyroidism

10. **The point prevalence of schizophrenia in people with learning disability is**
    A. 1%
    B. 20%
    C. 3%
    D. 15%
    E. 10%

11. **An 18-year-old man with learning disability has ectopia lentis, fair hair, long thin limbs, and osteoporosis. The most likely diagnosis is**
    A. Phenylketonuria
    B. Homocystinuria
    C. Marfan syndrome
    D. Tay Sach's disease
    E. Fragile X syndrome

12. **The social approach of providing a pattern of life as ordinary as possible for the learning disabled population is called**
    A. Community rehabilitation
    B. Eugenics
    C. Normalization
    D. Reality orientation
    E. Standardization

13. **The proportion of the learning disabled population with an IQ in the range 50–70 is**
    A. 10%
    B. 2%
    C. 4%
    D. 85%
    E. 40%

14. **A landmark epidemiological study in child psychiatry is the Isle of Wight study in the UK. What was the nature of the original sample first studied?**
    A. A sub-sample of all children aged 5–13
    B. Every other child aged 5–17
    C. A sub-sample of all children aged 9–15
    D. All children aged 9–11
    E. Every other child aged 9–12

15. **The point prevalence of any ICD-10 disorders in 5- to 15-year-old children is estimated to be around**
    A. 1%
    B. 5%
    C. 10%
    D. 20%
    E. 25%

16. **Comparable male and female prevalence rates are found for which of the following psychiatric disorders in children?**
    A. Eating disorders
    B. Hyperactivity disorders
    C. Nocturnal enuresis
    D. Selective mutism
    E. Tourette's syndrome

17. **According to the Isle of Wight study the ratio of boys to girls with conduct disorder is**
    A. 4:1
    B. 2:1
    C. 1:2
    D. 10:1
    E. Conduct disorder was not diagnosed in girls

18. **Reactive attachment disorder is a recognized category in both ICD-10 and DSM-IV. Which of the following criteria used for diagnosing this condition is mentioned in DSM-IV but not ICD-10?**
    A. Markedly disturbed inappropriate social relatedness
    B. The disturbance does not meet the criteria for pervasive developmental disorder
    C. Onset before 5 years of age
    D. A history of significant neglect
    E. The disturbance in relationships is a direct result of abnormal care-giving

19. **The term frozen watchfulness is used in description of which of the following psychiatric conditions?**
    A. Inhibited reactive attachment disorder
    B. Autism
    C. Selective mutism
    D. Social anxiety disorder
    E. Post-traumatic stress disorder

20. **Which of the following best defines the diagnosis of specific reading disorder when assessed using psychometric measures of reading age?**
    A. Reading age is below the 10th percentile of the peers
    B. Reading age is one standard deviation below the expected
    C. Reading age is two standard deviations below the expected
    D. Reading age is three standard deviations below the expected
    E. Reading age is below the 20th percentile of the peers

21. **A 10-year-old boy makes repeated errors in reading and spelling with substitutions and omissions of letters. He is slow in reading with considerable hesitations. All of the following features are expected in this child except**
    A. Minor neurological abnormalities
    B. Socially disadvantaged home setting
    C. Lower rates of conduct disorder
    D. Higher rates of similar problems in the family
    E. Higher rates of emotional problems

22. **The most consistent genetic locus implicated in specific reading disorder is**
    A. Chromosome 6p
    B. Chromosome 9p
    C. Chromosome 12p
    D. Chromosome 4p
    E. Chromosome 1p

23. **Which of the following is a common condition in childhood that is not listed as a separate disorder in ICD-10?**
    A. Sleepwalking
    B. Stuttering
    C. Tic disorder
    D. Autism
    E. Sibling rivalry

24. **All of the following are recognized associations with specific reading disorder except**
    A. Difficulty in visual scanning
    B. Right – left confusion
    C. Age related spontaneous resolution
    D. Higher rates in epileptic children
    E. Deterioration in acquired language skills

25. **The prevalence of autism is estimated to be around**
    A. 6 per 1000 children
    B. 10 per 1000 children
    C. 1 per 10000 children
    D. 1 per 1000 children
    E. 1 per 100000 children

26. **Which of the following condition is associated with intractable epilepsy, autism-like features and skin lesions in children?**
    A. Congenital hypothyroidism
    B. Fragile X syndrome
    C. Tuberous sclerosis
    D. Foetal alcohol syndrome
    E. Benzodiazepine use in pregnancy

27. During clinical assessment of temper tantrums in a child the most important initial step is to

   A. Assess IQ of the child
   B. Elicit family history of temper tantrums
   C. Explore parental limit setting behaviour
   D. Explore suicidal ideas in the child
   E. Record family history of criminality

28. Controlled evaluations of family therapy in child psychiatric conditions have demonstrated significant beneficial effects for which of the following?

   A. Anorexia nervosa in adolescents
   B. Pervasive developmental disorder
   C. Hyperkinetic disorder
   D. School refusal
   E. Specific reading disorder

29. Family therapy is indicated in all of the following situations in child psychiatry except

   A. The child's symptoms are an expression of family's malfunction
   B. Individual therapy for the child is not effective
   C. Family difficulties are identified during the course of another therapy
   D. The marriage of the child's parents is breaking up
   E. Family spontaneously seeks the therapy

30. Which of the following scales is used as a screening instrument to identify possible developmental difficulties that need further assessment?

   A. British ability scales
   B. Denver screening test
   C. Neale analysis
   D. Stanford Binet test
   E. Weschler scale

31. The prevalence of bullying is estimated to be around

   A. 1–2% of children, at least once a week
   B. 2–8% children, at least once a month
   C. 2–8% children, at least once a day
   D. 12–18% children, at least once a week
   E. 2–8% children, at least once a week

32. Which of the following attachment pattern is the best predictor of future development of conduct problems?

   A. Disorganized
   B. Secure
   C. Ambivalent
   D. Resistant
   E. None of the above

33. **Ainsworth's strange situation procedure is usually used to study patterns of attachment in which of the following the age groups?**
    A. 30–36 months
    B. 12–18 months
    C. 3–6 months
    D. 24–36 months
    E. 18–30 months

34. **Blood levels of which of the following substances has been adversely associated with IQ of a child?**
    A. Iron
    B. Lead
    C. Lithium
    D. Magnesium
    E. Sodium

35. **The multiaxial system of classification for child and adolescent psychiatric disorders in ICD-10 consists of**
    A. three axes
    B. four axes
    C. five axes
    D. six axes
    E. seven axes

36. **The average age range of attaining physical changes of puberty in boys is**
    A. 10–12 years
    B. 11–13 years
    C. 13–16 years
    D. 16–19 years
    E. 9–10 years

37. **The proportion of children with childhood autism that show improvement by the age of 6 years is**
    A. 1–2%
    B. 5–8%
    C. 8–10%
    D. 25–30%
    E. 10–20%

38. **In families with one autistic child, the risk of a further autistic child is about**
    A. 1–1.5%
    B. 3–5%
    C. 10–15%
    D. 30–35%
    E. 50–60%

39. **The estimated heritability of attention deficit hyperactivity disorder (ADHD) is around**
    A. 10%
    B. 25%
    C. 33%
    D. 50%
    E. 70%

40. **All of the following factors predict poor outcome in conduct disorders except**
    A. Late-onset conduct problems
    B. Multiple and varied symptoms and behaviours
    C. Parental psychiatric disorder
    D. Parental criminality
    E. Associated hyperactivity

41. **Among the juvenile delinquent population, the most commonly committed offence is**
    A. Sexual assault
    B. Homicide
    C. Fraud
    D. Property offences
    E. Offences related to terrorism

42. **All of the following are associated with higher rates of nocturnal enuresis except**
    A. Family history of enuresis
    B. Male sex
    C. Overcrowded home
    D. Rigid parental toilet training
    E. Stressful life events

43. **The most common form of medically unexplained symptom complained by children is**
    A. Recurrent chest pain
    B. Recurrent headaches
    C. Recurrent fever
    D. Recurrent memory loss
    E. Recurrent palpitations

44. **A psychometric test involves experimental creation of a situation in which a test person has to distinguish his or her own knowledge of a hidden object from the knowledge of the others. This test is called**
    A. Sally & Anne Task
    B. Draw a Person Test
    C. Thematic Apperception Test
    D. Lucy & Linda Task
    E. Rorschach's test

45. **Which is the most consistently identified abnormality in neurobiological studies of autism?**
    A. Elevated urinary dopamine metabolites
    B. Elevated urinary metanephrines
    C. Raised cerebrospinal fluid (CSF) 5-HIAA
    D. Raised serotonin blood levels
    E. Low platelet MAO levels

46. **Comparing autism and Asperger's syndrome, which of the following is true?**
    A. Head growth deceleration is seen in autism but not Asperger's syndrome
    B. High male: female ratio is seen in Asperger's syndrome but not autism
    C. Seizures are more common in Asperger's syndrome than autism
    D. Social skills before the age of 3 is normal in Asperger's syndrome
    E. The degree of learning disability is milder in Asperger's syndrome

47. **All of the following symptoms are more common in depression associated with learning disability than in those of normal intelligence except**
    A. Irritability
    B. Sleep disturbances
    C. Tearfulness
    D. Decline in social skills
    E. Hypochondriasis

48. **A residential care home has 12 residents with learning disability. The nurses at the care home want to use a screening instrument at regular intervals to detect likely mental health problems among the residents. Which of the following would be most suitable?**
    A. Psychiatric Assessment Schedule for Adults with Developmental Disabilities
    B. Diagnostic interview schedule
    C. Camberwell Assessment of Need for Adults with Developmental and Intellectual Disabilities
    D. Schedule for Clinical Assessment in Neuropsychiatry
    E. General Health Questionnaire

49. **An 8-year-old boy suffers from episodes of sudden but brief flexion of neck and trunk and flexion of legs at the hips since the age of one. He has severe mental retardation. Which of the following EEG pattern is most likely in this boy?**
    A. Diffuse triphasic delta waves
    B. Flat EEG trace
    C. Background high voltage slow waves intermixed with asynchronous spikes in both hemispheres
    D. Low voltage EEG with no spikes
    E. Periodic 3/second spikes

50. **Which of the following is true with respect to the use of medications to treat behavioural problems in learning disabled individuals?**
    A. Antidepressants are the most effective intervention
    B. Haloperidol is the most effective intervention
    C. Low dose lorazepam has the best evidence base
    D. Placebo effect surpasses active medications
    E. Risperidone is more effective in high doses

1. E.   One of the most common causes of death in Down's syndrome is congenital heart disease. Common phenotypic features seen in children with Down's syndrome include brachycephaly, broad hands, single palmar crease, epicanthal folds, clinodactyly of fifth finger, flat nasal bridge, and wide gap between first and second toes, hypotonia with lax ligaments, short stature, and mental retardation. In addition, children may have congenital heart defects such as ventricular septal defect, duodenal atresia at birth, and increased incidence of leukaemia in childhood. Atlantoaxial subluxation may occur in children with Down's syndrome, leading to spinal cord compression. The signs and symptoms of hypothyroidism can develop slowly over time and can be difficult to discriminate from those of Down's syndrome itself. No differences have been found in terms of age of onset of the physical features of puberty in adolescent girls and boys with Down's syndrome compared with general population trends. In men, reproductive capacity appears to be diminished, but women with Down's syndrome are able to bear children.

Roizen NJ and Patterson D. Down's syndrome. *Lancet* 2003; **361**: 1281–1289.

2. A.   Children with Down's syndrome are known to be gentle, mild mannered, and easygoing. It is reported that emotional and behavioural problems are less frequent than other forms of learning disabilities. Medical causes must be ruled out before considering a *de novo* psychiatric explanation for behavioural and emotional problems. The dual diagnoses of Down's syndrome and autism has been recognized for some time, with recent reports quoting 7% of Down's syndrome children having autism. Puri *et al.* (2001) showed in a study of 68 adults with Down's syndrome that individuals aged over 45 with a history of seizures were significantly more likely to develop Alzheimer's dementia; nearly 84% of demented individuals with Down's syndrome developed seizures. This is far higher than the rate of seizures found in Alzheimer's dementia without Down's syndrome (10%) and Down's syndrome without dementia (8%). Early-onset seizures in Down's syndrome seem to be unrelated to Alzheimer's type of pathology.

Puri BK, Ho KW and Singh I. Age of seizure onset in adults with Down's syndrome. *International Journal of Clinical Practice* 2001; **55**: 442–444.
Gelder MG, *et al.* eds. *Shorter Oxford Textbook of Psychiatry,* 5th edn. Oxford University Press, 2006, p. 717.

3. A.   EO Lewis suggested the distinction between subcultural learning disability and biological learning disability in 1933. 'Subcultural mental handicap' refers to the lower extreme variant of IQ distribution seen in the population. The biological or pathological type is seen to be evenly distributed across all social classes, whereas the subcultural type is often seen in social class V and associated with mild rather than profound disability. Kraeplin is associated with dementia praecox, and French psychiatrist Benoit Morel is associated with the theory of degeneration in schizophrenia. Kanner is associated with infantile autism.

Blackie J, Forrest A and Witcher G. Subcultural mental handicap. *British Journal of Psychiatry* 1975; **127**: 535–539.

4. E. The diagnostic criteria for foetal alcohol syndrome includes confirmed maternal alcohol exposure in addition to evidence of characteristic facial anomalies such as short palpebral fissures and abnormalities in the premaxillary zone, including flat upper lip, cleft palate, flattened philtrum, and flat midface. Evidence of growth retardation includes low birthweight for gestational age or decelerating weight gain over time not due to undernutrition. Features suggestive of neurodevelopmental abnormalities such as decreased cranial size at birth, structural brain abnormalities (e.g. microcephaly, partial or complete agenesis of the corpus callosum, cerebellar hypoplasia), and neurological signs (impaired fine motor skills, neurosensory hearing loss, poor tandem gait, poor eye–hand coordination) are also included in the diagnostic criteria. Congenital cataract is not suggestive of foetal alcohol syndrome; in infants with cataract, other explanations for developmental problems such as toxoplasmosis, congenital rubella, or metabolic syndromes must be sought.

Autti-Ramo I. Foetal alcohol syndrome – a multifaceted condition. *Developmental Medicine and Child Neurology* 2002; **44**: 141–144.

5. C. Subcultural learning disability refers to the lower extreme variant of IQ distribution seen in the population and it often seen in social class V and associated with mild rather than profound disability. Many family members of individuals with subcultural learning disability may also have borderline IQ, probably due to the effects of shared environment and social influences. In contrast, the biological or pathological type is seen to be evenly distributed across all social classes. Dysmophic features are more likely to be seen in those with a biological cause of learning disability with syndromic presentation being noted. Subcultural learning disability suggests the concept of a psychosocial causation (e.g. physical and emotional neglect). This is controversial.

Semple DM, *et al.* eds. *Oxford Handbook of Psychiatry,* 1st edn. Oxford University Press 2005, p. 687.

6. C. Smith–Magenis syndrome has a prevalence of 1 : 500 000. It is caused by a microdeletion on the short arm of chromosome 17p11·2. The degree of intellectual impairment is usually variable. The phenotype includes bradydactyly, a broad, flat face, hoarse voice, and a characteristic fleshy upper lip, although these features may be very subtle. Prominent autistic features, hyperactivity (in 75%), inattention, and self-injury (in 70%) such as head banging, nail pulling, and hand biting, are seen. Nocturnal and diurnal enuresis may also be present. Sleep is characterized by reduced or absent REM phase. Trisomy 21 refers to Down's syndrome. 7q11 deletion in the elastin gene can result in Williams syndrome, which is characterized by hyperactivity, 'cocktail party speech', and supravalvular aortic stenosis. Hypoxanthine guanine phosphoribosyltransferase deficiency can result in Lesch Nyhan syndrome with severe self-mutilation, aggression, and hyperuricaemia. Trisomy 13 syndrome is also known as Patau's syndrome and can be of three types: full trisomy, mosaic pattern type, and translocation type. All survivors have profound mental retardation.

Lask B, Taylor S and Nunn K, eds. *Practical Child Psychiatry: The Clinician's Guide.* BMJ Publishing, 2003, p. 161.

7. D. Autism is a disorder with lifelong disability. About 70% of autistic individuals have an IQ in the learning disability range. In autism, IQ has been shown to be the most powerful predictor of outcome. A distinctive cognitive profile characterized by strong visuospatial skills and poor abstract ability has been noted. A small proportion of autistic children may have islets of special abilities and are dubbed as 'autistic savants'. The presence of communicative speech by the age of 5 years is another important predictor of positive outcome.

Lask B, Taylor S, Nunn K, eds. *Practical Child Psychiatry: The Clinician's Guide.* BMJ Publishing, 2003, p. 178.
Volkmar FR, Pauls D. Autism. *Lancet* 2003; **362**: 1133–1141.

8. D. In a sample of more than 2500 boys born in 1981, details of bullying and victimization were gathered when the boys were 8 years old. Between the ages of 18 and 23, information about psychiatric disorders was collected from a registry. The boys could be classified into those who bully others, those who are frequently victimized, and those who bully others and are victimized frequently. Frequent bullying-only status predicted antisocial personality and substance abuse; frequent victimization-only status predicted anxiety disorder, whereas frequent bully–victim status predicted antisocial personality and anxiety disorder. Frequent bully–victims were at particular risk of adverse long-term outcomes compared with either pure bullies or pure victims.

Sourander A, Jensen P, Ronning JA, et al. What is the early adulthood outcome of boys who bully or are bullied in childhood? The Finnish 'From a Boy to a Man' study. *Pediatrics* 2007; **120**: 397–404.

9. B. Fragile X syndrome is the most common known inherited cause of learning disability. It affects 1:3600 boys and 1:6000 girls. Thirty per cent of individuals affected by fragile X have autistic features. Nearly 20% have epilepsy too. 1 in 300 women and 1 in 800 men are carriers of fragile X mutation. Although Down's syndrome is a more common cause of learning disability, it is mostly sporadic and not inherited in the strict sense.

Gelder MG, et al. eds. *Shorter Oxford Textbook of Psychiatry,* 5th edn. Oxford University Press, 2006, p. 714.

10. C. The point prevalence of schizophrenia is estimated to be between 3% and 4% in the learning-disabled population compared with 1% in the general population. Schizophrenia cannot be reliably diagnosed below an IQ of approximately 45. Often in clinical practice, if there is evidence of delusions or hallucinations in those with profound learning disability, a diagnosis of psychosis not otherwise specified is used. Despite this the rate of schizophrenia is significantly higher among the population with learning disability. This increase is seen despite the overall rate of psychiatric illness among adults with mild to moderate learning disability being similar to that in the general adult population without learning disability. The reason for this increased comorbidity is unclear, and common underlying brain damage that could cause both learning disability and schizophrenia cannot be ruled out.

Deb S, Thomas M and Bright C. Mental disorder in adults with intellectual disability. 1. Prevalence of functional psychiatric illness among a community-based population aged between 16 and 64 years. *Journal of Intellectual Disability Research* 2001; **45**: 495–505.

11. B. Homocystinuria is a metabolic disorder characterized by an increased blood and urine concentration of amino acid homocysteine. Clinical features resemble Marfan syndrome; patients have ectopia lentis, chest and spinal deformities similar to Marfan syndrome. But changes in hair colour, osteoporosis, arterial and venous thrombosis, and learning disabilities are generally absent in patients with Marfan syndrome.

Gelder MG, et al., eds. *Shorter Oxford Textbook of Psychiatry,* 5th edn. Oxford University Press, 2006, p. 715.

12. C. In the past, learning disability has been a cause for social rejection, with prejudiced labels such as 'degeneracy' associated with it. The so-called degenerates were isolated from the community, leading to the establishment of large mental institutions. The principle of normalization is seen by many as a reaction to the dehumanizing policies of the past. Normalization promotes independence and autonomy while making it possible for people with learning disabilities to have an ordinary life with the same choices and opportunities as everyone else. This shifts the focus from 'disability' to 'differences in ability'.

Gelder MG, et al., eds. *Shorter Oxford Textbook of Psychiatry* 5th edn. Oxford University Press, 2006, p. 722.

13. D.   Nearly 85% of those with learning disability have an IQ in the range 50–70 (mild learning disability). Of the rest, nearly 10% have moderate learning disability with an IQ in the range 35–50 and around 5% have an IQ in the severe/profound learning disability range (less than 35).

Gelder MG, et al., eds. *Shorter Oxford Textbook of Psychiatry*, 5th edn. Oxford University Press, 2006, p. 708.

14. D.   Major epidemiological work in child psychiatry started with the Isle of Wight surveys between 1964 and 1974. The Isle of Wight surveys had a two-phase design, with a systematic questionnaire screening a large sample, followed by in-depth assessments of a sub-sample selected according to the results of screening. Multiple informants were used in both phases. All 9- to 11-year-old children attending state schools on the island were included in the primary survey. A 4-year follow-up was carried out for children identified with psychiatric problems when they were approximately 14 years old.

Rutter M. Isle of Wight revisited: twenty-five years of child psychiatric epidemiology. *Journal of the American Academy of Child and Adolescent Psychiatry* 1989; **28**: 633–653.

15. C.   Numerous cross-sectional epidemiological surveys have confirmed that psychopathology in young people is common, with most studies estimating the prevalence to be between 10% and 20%. In a study that included more than 10 000 children, overall rates of psychiatric disorders in 5- to 15-year-old children in UK was estimated to be around 9.5%. A review of 49 surveys worldwide indicated an average point prevalence of 12.9% for psychiatric disorders in children. Emotional disturbances and behavioural disorders are equally common. Only a small proportion – between 10% and 30% – of children with a psychiatric disorder make contact with specialist mental health services.

Martin A, Volkmar FR, eds. *Lewis's Child and Adolescent Psychiatry: A Comprehensive Textbook*, 4th edn. Lippincott Williams and Wilkins, 2007, p. 164.

16. D.   Pervasive developmental disorders such as autism and Asperger's syndrome are more common in boys. Attention deficit hyperactivity disorder, tic disorders, oppositional defiance, and conduct disorders are also seen more often in boys than in girls. The rate of depression seems equal between both sexes before puberty. School refusal and selective mutism are also equally common in both boys and girls. Depression after puberty, specific phobia, eating disorders, and enuresis in daytime are more common in girls. Nocturnal enuresis in older children is more prevalent in boys.

Gelder MG, et al., eds. *Shorter Oxford Textbook of Psychiatry*, 5th edn. Oxford University Press, 2006, p. 651 (see Table 24.2).

17. A.   Conduct disorders are four times more common in boys than in girls according to the Isle of Wight study. Girls are more prone to use verbal and relational violence, such as exclusion from groups and character defamation, than the physical attacks seen in boys. Consequently, girls are violent in a way that can be difficult to document and to describe as conduct disorder symptoms; this may be a reason for under-diagnosis of conduct issues in girls.

Gelder MG, et al., eds. *Shorter Oxford Textbook of Psychiatry*, 5th edn. Oxford University Press, 2006, p. 650.

18. E. The core features of reactive attachment disorder (RAD) are preserved across both diagnostic nosologies, ICD and DSM. But the focus on subtypes and emphasis on the pathogenic nature of care giving are different. The DSM-IV includes inhibited and disinhibited types of RAD. In ICD-10, the term reactive attachment disorder stands for inhibited type, while disinhibited attachment disorder is separately defined. Both ICD and DSM endorse problems of social relatedness in RAD. Age of onset criteria (before 5 years) and exclusion of pervasive developmental disorders are common for both nosologies. In addition, DSM-IV also requires the presence of a known history of grossly pathogenic care, suggesting a causal link. Children with the disinhibited subtype may appear indiscriminately social.

Gelder MG, et al., eds. *Shorter Oxford Textbook of Psychiatry*, 5th edn. Oxford University Press, 2006, p. 667.

19. A. The term 'frozen watchfulness' describes an alertness or even hypervigilance that is maintained despite an overall inhibition of motor activity that may include mutism. Reactive attachment disorder (RAD) is associated with markedly disturbed and developmentally inappropriate social relatedness beginning before age 5 years. It commonly presents as persistent failure to initiate or respond to most social interactions. The responses can be excessively inhibited, hypervigilant, or highly ambivalent and contradictory. This is associated with avoidance of resistance to comforting or exhibiting a frozen watchfulness. This type of RAD is called the inhibited type. In disinhibited type, diffuse attachments manifested by indiscriminate sociability with marked inability to exhibit appropriately selective attachments are seen. This frozen watchfulness is different from aloofness seen in autism or dissociative features seen in PTSD. Frozen watchfulness is also seen in young victims of physical abuse.

Hornor G. Reactive Attachment Disorder. *Journal of Pediatric Health Care* 2008; **22**: 234–239.

20. C. According to current classificatory systems, a learning disorder such as specific reading disorder can be diagnosed when the child achieves substantially lower than expected scores on individually administered, standardized tests of components of learning (reading, mathematics, or written expression) for a given age, schooling, and level of intelligence. Thus an explicit reference to psychometric assessments is made when diagnosing learning disorders. But a specific guideline as to the statistical meaning of being substantially below the expected norm is not clearly delineated in DSM IV. Nevertheless, ICD-10 states a score that is at least 2 standard errors of prediction below the expected value as diagnostic criteria for specific developmental disorders of scholastic skills.

Gelder MG, et al., eds. *Shorter Oxford Textbook of Psychiatry*, 5th edn. Oxford University Press, 2006, p. 667.

21. C. This child is most likely having specific reading disorder. This is associated with higher prevalence of emotional disturbances and conduct disorder. It is more often seen in boys than girls. Minor soft neurological signs are frequently seen in children with this disorder, suggesting a neural developmental abnormality.

Martin A and Volkmar FR, eds. *Lewis's Child and Adolescent Psychiatry: A Comprehensive Textbook*, 4th edn. Lippincott Williams and Wilkins, 2007, p.413.

22. A. Specific reading disorder is regarded to have significant genetic aetiology, with multiple genes contribute to the biological risk factor. The candidate regions are abbreviated as DYX1 to DYX9 on chromosomes 15q, 6p, 2p, 6q, 3cen, 18p, 11p, 1p, and Xq, respectively. Of these, the most consistent findings seem to be the role of chromosome 6.

Gelder MG, et al., eds. *Shorter Oxford Textbook of Psychiatry*, 5th edn. Oxford University Press, 2006, p. 668.

23. B.   Among the specific disorders of psychological development listed in the question, stuttering is not a separate diagnostic category in the current ICD-10, Chapter V. Stuttering has a high incidence between second and fourth years of life affecting 4% to 5% of the population with nearly equal sex ratio at the start. Normal developmental dysfluencies tend to occur in the larger linguistic units such as words, phrases, and sentences. In stutterers this occurs in repetitions of syllables and prolongation of sounds. Recovery usually occurs by adolescence and is more likely in girls; nearly 1 in 30 children have stuttering though only 1% of adolescents show stuttering. A familial component is noted in stuttering - the risk in first-degree relatives being more than three times the population risk.

Sleepwalking, sibling rivalry disorder, tic disorder and autism are definite diagnostic categories in ICD-10.

Martin A and Volkmar FR, eds. *Lewis's Child and Adolescent Psychiatry: A Comprehensive Textbook*, 4th edn. Lippincott Williams and Wilkins, 2007, p. 424.

24. E.   Deterioration of already acquired language skills is not seen in specific reading disorder or dyslexia. Neurodevelopmental basis for dyslexia is suggested by the similarity of certain symptoms in dyslexic children and the neurological syndrome of `visual word blindness' that results from damage to the left inferior parieto-occipital region (more specifically, the left angular gyrus). This region is speculated to have a role in processing the optic images of letters; damage to this region may lead to defects in visual scanning. It is also noted that dyslexic children have poor or delayed brain lateralization, especially for language. The high incidence of left-handers, right-left confusion and the mirror-writing phenomenon noted in dyslexia can be considered as indirect support to this notion. Epileptic children may have higher incidence of dyslexia. General improvement with age suggests a brain maturational delay in the aetiology of dyslexia.

Gelder MG, *et al.*, eds. *Shorter Oxford Textbook of Psychiatry*, 5th edn. Oxford University Press, 2006, p. 669.
Habib M. The neurological basis of developmental dyslexia: an overview and working hypothesis. *Brain* 2000; **123**: 2373–2399.

25. D.   Preliminary surveys regarding epidemiology of autism reported 2 -5 cases of autism per 10 000 children. Wide variations have been reported in later studies ranging from 0·7 to 21 per 10 000 children (median 4–5 per 10 000). At present, at least one in 1000 children are estimated to have autism. Differences in methodology of surveys and wide variations in the definition of autism are the main reasons behind such variations. It is noted that boys have three-to-four-fold higher rates of autism.

Volkmar FR and Pauls D. Autism. *Lancet* 2003; **362**: 1133–1141.

26. C.   Tuberous sclerosis is an autosomal dominant genetic multisystem disorder characterised by widespread hamartomas in the brain, heart, skin, eyes, kidney, lung, and liver. Most features of tuberous sclerosis become evident only in childhood after 3 years of age. The affected genes *TSC1* and *TSC* encode for proteins hamartin and tuberin respectively. Epilepsy is seen in 60–80% tuberous sclerosis cases and is thought to be secondary to changes of GABA receptors in dysplastic neurons, and enhanced excitation via glutamate receptors in cortical hamartomas. The epilepsy is generally of an early onset and is often intractable in severity. Hypomelanotic macules are the most common dermatological manifestation; they are seen in 90–98% of patients with tuberous sclerosis.

Curatolo P, Bombardieri R and Jozwiak S. Tuberous sclerosis. *Lancet*; **372**: 657–668.

27. C.   Temper tantrums are common in children between the ages of 18 months and 4 years. Tantrum behaviours range from simple crying to dramatic attention-seeking events such as breath holding and head banging in otherwise normal children. Often parents may be reinforcing tantrum behaviour without knowledge and may have an inconsistent approach to discipline and limit setting. Hence the first step in assessment of a family with a child throwing frequent temper tantrums is discovering why parents are not able to set consistent limits.
Gelder MG, et al., eds. *Shorter Oxford Textbook of Psychiatry*, 5th edn. Oxford University Press, 2006, p. 666.

28. A.   The strongest evidence base for using family therapy exists for anorexia nervosa in adolescents. By the end of family therapy sessions more than 50% adolescent girls reach a healthy weight; it is estimated that more than 60% achieve recovery on follow up. Encouraging parents to take an active role is seen as a vital component; not involving the parents in the treatment leads to the worst outcome and may delay recovery considerably. Other conditions with evidence base for the use of systemic family therapy include childhood mood disorders, substance abuse and conduct problems in children.
Gelder MG, et al., eds. *Shorter Oxford Textbook of Psychiatry*, 5th edn. Oxford University Press, 2006, p. 663.
Asen E. Outcome research in family therapy. *Advances in Psychiatric Treatment* 2002 2002; **8**: 230–238.

29. D.   Family therapy considers the symptoms in a child to be expression of family dysfunction. It can be used if such dysfunctions are evident during assessment, or if individual therapy fails or to manage family difficulties arising in the course of other treatments. As in other forms of psychotherapy, no blanket indications and contraindications can be listed for family therapy. But there are some instances in which therapists do not advise the family to undergo therapy. In families where parental marital relationship is breaking down, highly fixed psychopathology that blocks any communication in family sessions and extreme schizoid or paranoid pathology are some of the instances where family therapy does not come as first choice of psychotherapy.
Gelder MG, et al., eds. *Shorter Oxford Textbook of Psychiatry*, 5th edn. Oxford University Press, 2006, p. 663.

30. B.   Denver developmental screening test can be applied from birth to 6 ½ years to identify delays in personal, language, motor and social development in children. It is purely a screening tool and any children identified to have developmental delays should undergo further assessment. Neale analysis of reading is a specific test of educational attainment (reading accuracy and comprehension). Stanford Binet test measures IQ using norms starting from age 2 to adulthood. Wechsler intelligence scale for children tests IQ for children between ages 6 – 14 years. A preschool and primary school version to test children aged 3 – 7 is also available. British ability scales are tests of intelligence covering varied areas such as speed of processing, spatial imagery, short term memory, perceptual matching and application of knowledge.
Gelder MG, et al., eds. *Shorter Oxford Textbook of Psychiatry*, 5th edn. Oxford University Press, 2006, p. 659.

31. E. A large survey in United Kingdom reported that 10% of pupils at a secondary school had been bullied during one term, with 2–8% (average 4%) reporting being bullied at least once a week. The commonest type of bullying is general name calling, followed by being hit, threatened, or having rumours spread about one. Bullying is more prevalent among boys; 30% of children do not tell anyone that they are bullied. This percentage is higher for boys and older children.

Gelder MG, et al., eds. *Shorter Oxford Textbook of Psychiatry*, 5th edn. Oxford University Press, 2006, p. 656.
http://www.nspcc.org.uk/Inform/resourcesforprofessionals/Statistics/KeyCPStats/10_wda48744. html (Accessed 14 March 2009).

32. A. Various aetiological contributors for conduct disorders include family stressors, parental discipline, child characteristics such as temperament or neurobiological problems and attachment relationships. Attachment behaviours include those infant behaviours that are activated by stress and that have as a goal the reduction of arousal and reinstatement of a sense of security. Such reinstatement is usually best achieved in infancy by close physical contact with a familiar caregiver. In addition to Ainsworth's initial description of secure, ambivalent and avoidant attachment patterns, Main and Solomon described a fourth infant attachment category called disorganized type. As many as 10 - 15% of children in some samples show disorganized type of attachment. Such disorganized attachment pattern presents with high levels of aggression, more externalizing and controlling behaviour in middle childhood. This is strongly related to aggressive disorders such as conduct disorder in childhood.

Lyons-Ruth K. Attachment relationships among children with aggressive behavior problems: the role of disorganized early attachment patterns. *Journal of Consulting and Clinical Psychology* 1996; **64**: 64–73.

33. B. Strange Situations procedure was initially employed by Mary Ainsworth to study attachment behaviours in children between ages 12 to 18 months. The experiment takes place in a room with a one-way mirror and attractive toys. The expected behaviour includes running around, clinging and reunion; so the children need to be somewhat mobile between ages 12 and 18 months.

Gelder MG, et al., eds. *Shorter Oxford Textbook of Psychiatry*, 5th edn. Oxford University Press, 2006, p. 656.

34. B. Lead is established to have neurotoxic effects on growing brain; blood lead concentrations above 10 µg per decilitre (0.483 µmol per litre) are associated with adverse intellectual functioning and social–behavioural conduct. A blood lead concentration of 10 µg per decilitre or higher is designated as a 'level of concern' by the World Health Organization. It is estimated that a loss of 7.4 IQ points takes place with a lifetime average blood lead concentration of up to 10 µg per decilitre.

Canfield RL, Henderson CR Jr, Cory-Slechta DA, et al. Intellectual Impairment in Children with Blood Lead Concentrations below 10 µg per decilitre. *New England Journal of Medicine* 2003; **348**: 1517–1526.

35. D. Multiaxial classification is very useful for child and adolescent psychiatric disorders due to the inherent complexity of information required in diagnosis and treatment. In the absence of a multiaxial system, certain conditions may easily get overlooked, such as the developmental learning disorders in a child with conduct problems. But the placement of certain disorders within a multiaxial framework may be problematic especially when the disorders have no specific aetiology and spans across multiple axes used in the classification. ICD-10 recommends six axes for diagnosing mental health problems in children. These include (1) psychiatric syndromes; (2) disorders of psychological development; (3) intellectual level; (4) medical conditions; (5) abnormal psychosocial situations; (6) global assessment of functioning. In contrast DSM-IV has five axes in total, as psychiatric symptoms and developmental disorders come under axis 1.

Gelder MG, *et al.*, eds. *Shorter Oxford Textbook of Psychiatry*, 5th edn. Oxford University Press, 2006, p. 649.

36. C. The average age at which physical changes of puberty occur is different for boys and girls. Tanner staging is often used to assess physical changes in puberty and stage 2 genital changes are used to define onset of puberty. It varies between 11 and 13 in girls, and 13 and 17 in boys. It must be noted that the criteria that more accurately reflect gonadal activity are breast development in girls and genital growth in boys. As these are difficult to ascertain, reliable measurement is not possible using observations of physical maturity; puberty as assessed by hormonal measurements of the hypothalamic pituitary gonadal axis is well established before physical signs appear.

Reiter EO. Have the onset and tempo of puberty changed? *Archives of Paediatric and Adolescent Medicine* 2001; **155**: 988–989.

37. E. By the age of 6 years, 10–20% of individuals with autism begin to improve. Eventually 15% of individuals achieve satisfactory self-sufficiency while another 20% manage with minimal periodic support. The remainder of at least 60% individuals does not achieve sufficient self sufficiency for an independent life. This outcome is variable according to degree of communicative language developed and IQ.

Gelder MG, *et al.*, eds. *Shorter Oxford Textbook of Psychiatry*, 5th edn. Oxford University Press, 2006, p. 674.

38. B. In families with one autistic child the risk of a further autistic child is around 3 – 5%. This sibling risk rate for autism denotes a tenfold increase over general population rates. Epidemiological studies of same sex autistic twins have identified around 60% monozygotic concordance while 0% for dizygotic twins. This difference becomes further pronounced when a broader autistic phenotype of related cognitive or social abnormalities are considered (92% of MZ pairs vs. 10% of DZ pairs). The risk to a monozygotic co-twin is estimated to be over 200 times the general population rate.

Baron-Cohen S. The cognitive neuroscience of autism. *Journal of Neurology, Neurosurgery, and Psychiatry* 2004; **75**: 945–948.

39. E.   The heritability of ADHD is estimated to be around 70%. Twin studies performed in several countries have shown that the average genetic contribution is 70–80% while non genetic variance contributes to 20–30%. It is also observed that 6% of adoptive parents of ADHD probands have ADHD compared to 18% of the biological parents of ADHD probands and 3% of the biological parents of the control probands. Siblings of children with hyperkinetic disorder have a 2–3 times greater risk of the disorder than siblings of normal controls.

Gelder MG, et al., eds. *Shorter Oxford Textbook of Psychiatry*, 5th edn. Oxford University Press, 2006, p. 677.

Wallis D, Russell HF, and Muenke M. Genetics of attention deficit/hyperactivity disorder. *Journal of Pediatric Psychology* 2008; **33**: 1085–1099.

40. A.   Childhood conduct disorder can continue as adult antisocial personality disorder. A wide range of other psychiatric disorders including substance abuse, major depression, psychosis and various adverse outcomes such as suicide, delinquency, educational difficulties and unemployment have been associated with conduct disorder. Evidence on prognosis of conduct disorder suggests dose-response relationship: The higher the number and variety of disruptive behaviours, the worse the adult outcomes. But most adolescents with conduct disorder do not develop antisocial personality in adulthood. Those who do not develop adverse outcomes as adults are most likely to have a late onset, adolescent-limited disorder rather than a life-course persistent problem with early onset. Other poor prognostic factors include severity, comorbid hyperactivity, pervasive behavioural disruption across varied settings and continuous exposure to risk factors.

Gelder MG, et al., eds. *Shorter Oxford Textbook of Psychiatry*, 5th edn. Oxford University Press, 2006, p. 679.

Martin A and Volkmar FR, eds. *Lewis's Child and Adolescent Psychiatry: A Comprehensive Textbook*, 4th edn. Lippincott Williams and Wilkins, 2007, p. 457.

41. D.   Among juvenile delinquents, the most common offences are against property. Boys are more delinquent than girls in a ratio of 4 to 11 delinquent boys for every delinquent girl. Among boys who get convicted only half get reconvicted. But most (nearly 75%) with repeated convictions become adult offenders.

Gelder MG, et al., eds. *Shorter Oxford Textbook of Psychiatry*, 5th edn. Oxford University Press, 2006, p. 680.

42. D.   Most enuretic children are free from psychiatric disorders. But the rate of psychiatric disorders is higher in enuretic than non-enuretic children. Children growing up in large families in overcrowded conditions have higher rate of enuresis. Stressful life events may form a starting point of secondary enuresis in children. Toilet training methods used by parents have not shown to be associated with enuresis. Enuresis tends to run in families; a positive family history can be related to positive treatment outcome. Many chromosomal loci have been identified - 13q, 12q, 8, and 22. Rarely some families show an autosomal dominant mode of transmission with penetrance above 90%.

Martin A and Volkmar FR, eds. *Lewis's Child and Adolescent Psychiatry: A Comprehensive Textbook*, 4th edn. Lippincott Williams and Wilkins, 2007, p.658.

43. B. Recurrent headaches are the most common somatic symptom with no medical explanation complained by children, followed by abdominal pain. 10 to 30% of children admit having frequent headaches (at least weekly) while 7 to 25% admit having abdominal pain. Chest pain is reported by approximately 10% of school aged children. At least 7.5% of children admit to other musculoskeletal pains. Chronic fatigue syndrome appears to be uncommon in children with estimated prevalence less than 1%.

Martin A, Volkmar FR, eds. *Lewis's Child and Adolescent Psychiatry: A Comprehensive Textbook,* 4th edn. Lippincott Williams and Wilkins, 2007, p. 636.

44. A. The Sally and Anne Task involves metarepresentation of another person's mental state. Two test characters Sally and Anne are shown in a picture. Sally leaves a toy at a place. Anne hides the toy at a different place in the absence of Sally. When Sally returns, where will she look for the toy - the place it was before she left the scene or the place where it had been moved by Anne? This requires a subject to distinguish his or her own knowledge that an object has been hidden by Anne in the absence of Sally from the knowledge of Sally. The test subject must be able to reflect Sally's mental state i.e. 'I know that she does not know where the object really is'. The Sally and Anne Test therefore tests understanding a first order false belief. As theory of mind does not develop fully before age 4, children under this age very often fail the test.

Brune M. 'Theory of Mind' in schizophrenia: a review of the literature. *Schizophrenia Bulletin* 2005; **31**: 21–42.

45. D. One of the most consistently observed biological findings in autism is increased serotonin levels in the blood, which is noted in 30–50% of children with autism. The high whole blood serotonin is also noted among family members of autistic patients. Essentially this whole blood level reflects platelet serotonin.

Connors SL, Matteson KJ, Sega GA, et al. Plasma serotonin in autism. *Pediatric Neurology* 2006; **35**: 182–186.

46. E. In both autism and Asperger's syndrome, males outnumber females. Communications skills are generally poor in autism, but fairly developed in Asperger's patients. Circumscribed narrow interests are usually severe in Asperger's syndrome. Seizures are uncommon in Asperger's patients while it is commoner in autism. Social skills are poorly developed in both autism and Asperger's disorder. IQ ranges from mild learning disability to normal level in Asperger's syndrome, while most patients with autism have low IQ. Head growth deceleration is not seen in both autism and Asperger's syndrome; it is a feature of Rett's disorder.

Volkmar FR and Pauls D. Autism. *Lancet* 2003; **362**: 1133–1141.

47. E. Though most symptoms of depression seen in learning disabled individuals are same as those seen in general population, certain differences exist. Cognitive syndrome of depression including memory disturbance and loss of concentration are often not detected. Similarly, guilt and recurrent thoughts of suicide are under-reported. But biological changes associated with depression such as psychomotor retardation, disturbed sleep, appetite and weight loss and diurnal variation in symptoms are more readily detected. Some symptoms may be more marked in depressed individuals with severe learning disability e.g. psychomotor agitation, irritability and behavioural disturbance. Decline in established activities of daily living and tearfulness may be signs of hidden depression in some patients. Hypochondriasis and other formed beliefs are rarely seen.

Prasher V. Presentation and management of depression in people with learning disability. *Advances in Psychiatric Treatment* 1999; **5**: 447–454.

48. A.   Measurement of psychopathology in people with learning disabilities is difficult. This issue is partly addressed by the Psychiatric Assessment Schedule for Adults with Developmental Disabilities (PAS–ADD) interview. A shorter version is also available and can be used as a screening tool by untrained people to identify clients with learning disabilities at risk of developing a psychiatric disorder. It contains 29 items concerning symptoms of psychiatric disorders, split into five scales that combine to produce three total scores: 1, affective/neurotic disorder; 2, possible organic disorder; and 3, psychotic disorder. Scores equal to or above specified thresholds indicate if a further assessment is necessary.

Sturmey P, Newton JT, Cowley A, *et al.* The PAS-ADD checklist: independent replication of its psychometric properties in a community sample. *British Journal of Psychiatry* 2005; **186**: 319–323.

49. C.   This child is most likely to have infantile spasms. This condition appears usually at the ages of 4 to 6 months. The spasms are a form of epilepsy and are characterised by sudden, brief flexion of neck and trunk, raising both arms forwards or and flexion of legs at the hips. A cry may be associated with the attack. The EEG is generally chaotic with slow waves of high voltage intermixed with asynchronous spikes in both hemispheres. This pattern of EEG findings is called hypsarrhythmia. Patients with infantile spasms limited to one side may have a surgically removable cortical dysplasia. Infantile spasms are also noted in infants with Down syndrome or tuberous sclerosis. The term West syndrome is applied to the triad of infantile spasms, hypsarrhythmia, and mental retardation.

Gelder MG, *et al.*, eds. *New Oxford Textbook of Psychiatry*. Oxford University Press 2000, pp. 1980–1981.

50. D.   Despite widespread use of antipsychotics to treat challenging behaviour in learning disabled adults, the evidence is scarce. 'Neuroleptics for Aggressive Challenging Behaviour in Intellectual Disability' (NACHBID) was a multicentre study that compared first-generation and second-generation antipsychotic drugs with placebo in patients with aggressive challenging behaviour. A reduction in aggression was noted with both antipsychotic treatments and placebo use after 4 weeks; the greatest response was with placebo. No differences between groups were observed in terms of aberrant behaviour, quality of life, general improvement or effect on carers. The combination of placebo effect, the psychological effect of a formal external intervention and/ or spontaneous resolution surpasses than the effect of medications.

Tyrer P, Oliver-Africano PC, Ahmed Z, *et al.* Risperidone haloperidol and placebo in the treatment of aggressive challenging behaviour in patients with intellectual disability: a randomised controlled trial. *Lancet* 2008; **371**: 57–63.

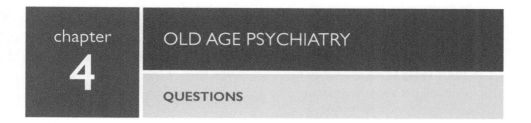

4

OLD AGE PSYCHIATRY

QUESTIONS

1. After a specific number of subcultivations in the laboratory, normal human cells undergo irreversible cessation of mitosis and enter a non-dividing state. This phenomenon is known as
   A. Programmed cell death
   B. Hayflick phenomenon
   C. Pruning
   D. G_0 phase arrest
   E. Cellular atrophy

2. The Hachinski Ischaemic Score is used to aid clinical differentiation of Alzheimer's dementia from vascular dementia. Which of the following clinical features support a diagnosis of Alzheimer's dementia rather than vascular dementia?
   A. Stepwise progression
   B. Fluctuating course
   C. Abrupt onset
   D. Early change in personality
   E. Nocturnal confusion

3. Which of the following statement regarding the assessment of activities of daily living (ADL) in elderly people is correct?
   A. ADL scales are used as outcome measures
   B. The Barthel index is a self-rating scale
   C. In dementia basic ADL are affected earlier than complex instrumental ADL
   D. None of the validated ADL scales depend on the patient's self-report
   E. The choice of ADL scale in a patient depends on the patient's gender

4. Schizophrenia-like psychosis is a prominent feature of which of the following dementing illnesses?
   A. Pick's disease
   B. Creutzfeldt–Jakob disease (CJD)
   C. Vascular dementia
   D. Huntington's dementia
   E. Lewy body dementia

5. **A 78-year-old man is treated with diazepam by his general practitioner for disabling anxiety related to a recent bereavement. The half-life of diazepam is most likely to be increased in this man due to**
   A. Increase in intestinal absorption
   B. Increase in oral bioavailability
   C. Increase in plasma protein binding
   D. Increase in volume of distribution
   E. Decrease in renal elimination

6. **Which of the following scales can be used to record the behavioural and psychological features associated with dementia in elderly people?**
   A. Neuropsychiatric inventory
   B. Schedule for clinical assessment in neuropsychiatry
   C. Bristol scale
   D. Cornell scale
   E. Abbreviated mental test

7. **Which of the following diagnostic tests has been most widely used to monitor treatment response in anticholinesterase trials for dementia?**
   A. Behaviour Pathology in Alzheimer's Disease rating scale
   B. Clock drawing test
   C. Alzheimer's disease assessment scale – cognitive section (ADAS-Cog)
   D. Mini Mental State Examination (MMSE)
   E. Magnetic resonance imaging (MRI) brain scan

8. **The average annual decline on the MMSE scores for patients with a natural course of Alzheimer's dementia is**
   A. 1–2 points/year
   B. 3–4 points/year
   C. 5–6 points/year
   D. 7–9 points/year
   E. 9–11 points/year

9. **Hyponatraemia is a troublesome side-effect of treating depression in elderly people. All of the following are true with regard to the above except**
   A. More common in males
   B. More frequent when diuretics are co-prescribed
   C. Often related to inappropriate ADH secretion
   D. Risk increases with increase in age
   E. Symptoms overlap with primary depressive features

10. **Presenilin mutations that are associated with early-onset Alzheimer's dementia are proposed to affect which of the following enzymes?**

    A. κ Secretase
    B. Tau phosphorylation enzymes
    C. α Secretase
    D. β Secretase
    E. γ Secretase

11. **Which of the following is an observational tool designed to evaluate the quality of care and well-being of people with dementia in formal care settings?**

    A. Bristol Scale
    B. Burden Interview
    C. Caregiver Burden Scale
    D. Clinical Dementia Rating (CDR)
    E. Dementia Care Mapping (DCM)

12. **A 67-year-old retired educational psychologist presents with forgetfulness. All of the following are features seen in mild cognitive impairment (MCI) except**

    A. Presence of subjective memory complaint
    B. Objective memory impairment for age
    C. Preserved general cognitive function
    D. Normal functional activities
    E. Presence of family history of dementia

13. **Lund–Manchester criteria are used in the diagnosis of which of the following conditions?**

    A. Alzheimer's dementia
    B. Vascular dementia
    C. Lewy body dementia
    D. Frontotemporal dementia
    E. Huntington's dementia

14. **All of the following are features of visual hallucinations reported in dementia of Lewy bodies except**

    A. The images are vivid
    B. The images are mostly grey or black and white
    C. Animate objects are often seen
    D. The images are usually three dimensional
    E. They predict better response to cholinesterase inhibitors

15. **Two patients are admitted to an inpatient unit for elderly people with movement disturbances. Patient A has a diagnosis of Parkinson's disease while patient B is diagnosed with dementia with Lewy bodies. Which of the following is correct with regard to the extrapyramidal symptoms in these conditions?**
    A. Patient A is more likely to have greater postural instability than patient B
    B. Patient A is more likely to have greater facial impassivity than patient B
    C. Patient A is more likely to have tremors than patient B
    D. Both patients will have similar profiles of extrapyramidal features
    E. Patient B is more likely to have prominent cerebellar signs

16. **Which of the following is associated with poor antidepressant response in geriatric depression?**
    A. Earlier age of onset
    B. Structural white matter abnormalities
    C. Enlarged cerebral ventricles
    D. Cingulate hyper-metabolism during depression
    E. Presence of somatic symptoms

17. **Which of the following present at the time of onset of depression predict greater risk of depressive relapse after treatment discontinuation in elderly patients with depression?**
    A. Depressive cognitions
    B. Presence of guilt
    C. Executive dysfunction
    D. Episodic memory loss
    E. Psychomotor retardation

18. **Secondary depression may be caused by physical illnesses in elderly people. Which of the following is correct with regard to depression and physical illness?**
    A. Primary depression is not diagnosed in the presence of chronic medical illnesses in elderly people
    B. Secondary depression is more common than primary depression in elderly people
    C. Subclinical hypothyroidism is more common among depressed than non-depressed elderly people
    D. Depression is two to three times more common in those with chronic medical illnesses
    E. Many apparent physical illnesses are found on investigation to be due to somatoform disorders

19. **Psychosis in elderly people may be due to dementia, Parkinson's disease, or schizophrenia. Which of the following is correct with respect to the clinical features of late-onset psychotic syndromes?**

    A. Hallucinations are more common than delusions in psychosis due to Alzheimer's disease
    B. Visual hallucination is the most common symptom in very late-onset schizophrenia
    C. Partition delusions are characteristic of psychosis associated with parkinsonism
    D. Negative symptoms are predominant in very late-onset schizophrenia
    E. Paranoid delusions are the most common symptoms in late-onset schizophrenia

20. **Which of the following forms of grief therapy treats unresolved grief as a form of phobic avoidance?**

    A. Guided mourning
    B. Supportive grief counselling
    C. Focused group therapy
    D. Interpersonal psychotherapy
    E. Debriefing

21. **When compared with those with late-onset depression, elderly individuals with early-onset depression have**

    A. Less frequent family history of mood disorders
    B. Higher prevalence of dementia
    C. More sensory impairment
    D. Greater enlargement of the lateral ventricles of the brain
    E. Less white matter hyperintensities

22. **The most effective psychological intervention to reduce depression and emotional burden in caregivers of people with dementia is**

    A. Psychoeducational intervention
    B. Group behavioural management
    C. Individual behavioural management
    D. Supportive psychotherapy
    E. Coping skills enhancement

23. **Which of the following methods of psychological management of neuropsychiatric symptoms of dementia uses materials such as old newspapers and household items to stimulate memories and enable people to share and value their experiences?**

    A. Reminiscence therapy
    B. Validation therapy
    C. Reality orientation therapy
    D. Cognitive stimulation therapy
    E. Snoezelen therapy

24. **A 72-year-old man presents with paranoid delusions and ideas of reference. The most common cause of new onset psychotic symptoms in this age group is**
    A. Parkinson-related psychosis
    B. Very late-onset schizophrenia
    C. Drug-induced psychosis
    D. Alzheimer's dementia
    E. Lewy body dementia

25. **According to the stage theory of grief, the earliest response after a natural death of a family member is**
    A. Numbness and disbelief
    B. Yearning and anxiety
    C. Anger
    E. Depressed mood
    F. Acceptance of the loss

26. **Memory complaints that do not qualify for a diagnosis of dementia are common in elderly people. All of the following are shown to predict conversion from mild cognitive impairment (MCI) to dementia except**
    A. Hippocampal atrophy
    B. Family history of Alzheimer's dementia (AD)
    C. Carers' reports of impaired daily function
    D. Significantly poor cognitive abilities
    E. Presence of sensory impairment

27. **The annual rate of progression from mild cognitive impairment (MCI) to dementia is estimated to be around**
    A. 10–15%
    B. 20–25%
    C. 30–35%
    D. 1–2%
    E. 4–5%

28. **Median survival from the time of diagnosis for patients with Alzheimer's dementia (AD) is**
    A. 1–3 years
    B. 3–5years
    C. 5–8 years
    D. 10–12 years
    E. 15–18 years

29. **Braak stages are used in neuropathological quantification of brain changes in Alzheimer's disease. Which of the following is the basis of Braak's stages?**

    A. Senile plaques
    B. Neuritic plaques
    C. Cortical atrophy
    D. Neurofibrillary tangles
    E. Hippocampal volume

30. **Many subtypes of vascular dementia have been identified. Which of the following refers to Binswanger's disease?**

    A. Attenuation of subcortical white matter causing cognitive impairment
    B. Basal ganglia infarct causing cognitive impairment
    C. Multiple cortical infarcts causing cognitive impairment
    D. Periventricular white matter infarcts causing cognitive impairment
    E. Single strategically placed infarct causing cognitive impairment

31. **The risk of developing late-onset Alzheimer's dementia in first-degree relatives of patients with late-onset Alzheimer's dementia compared with controls is**

    A. 5 times higher
    B. 3 times higher
    C. 10 times higher
    D. No higher than the general population
    E. 16 times higher

32. **In CJD pathological study of brain tissue shows spongiosis with neuronal loss, gliosis, and amyloid plaques. These amyloid plaques contain**

    A. Synuclein
    B. Immunoglobulin
    C. Prion protein
    D. Amylin
    E. Presenilin

33. **Pulvinar sign is a MRI finding in which of the following conditions?**

    A. Huntington's dementia
    B. Variant CJD (vCJD)
    C. Lewy body dementia
    D. Subdural haematoma
    E. Extradual haemorrhage

34. **The most prevalent neurotic disorder among elderly people above the age of 65 is**

    A. Phobic disorders
    B. Obsessive compulsive disorder
    C. Generalized anxiety disorder
    D. Panic disorder
    E. Post-traumatic stress disorder

35. **Suicide is a significant risk when treating elderly patients with mental health problems. Compared with suicides in younger adults, older patients who kill themselves are**
    A. More likely to enter into suicide pacts
    B. More likely to be known to mental health services
    C. Less likely to suffer from depression
    D. More likely to be females
    E. More likely to have a treatment history for psychiatric complaints

36. **All of the following are necessary to establish the competence to make a will except**
    A. The person should know what the act of making a will means
    B. The person should have a broad understanding of the extent of his/her estate
    C. The person should know who might have claims on his/her possessions
    D. The person should not have a disorder affecting his/her mind
    E. The person should not be under any undue influence

37. **Compared with mania at younger age of onset, late-onset mania in elderly people is characterized by**
    A. Stronger genetic loading
    B. Lesser frequency of cerebral pathology
    C. Higher rates in women
    D. Higher admixture of depressive features
    E. Lesser risk of subsequent depressive episode on recovery

38. **Which of the following antidementia drugs acts directly on nicotinic receptors to increase cholinergic neurotransmission?**
    A. Memantine
    B. Donepezil
    C. Rivastigmine
    D. Galantamine
    E. Tacrine

39. **The plasma half-life of memantine is approximately**
    A. 2–4 hours
    B. 30–90 minutes
    C. 60–80 hours
    D. 24–48 hours
    E. 2–3 weeks

40. **The anticholinesterase agent with least drop-out rates in longitudinal trials is**
    A. Galantamine
    B. Tacrine
    C. Donepezil
    D. Rivastigmine
    E. All available agents have similar drop-out rates

41. In the pharmacological management of delirium, haloperidol is the preferred agent from the available antipsychotic drugs. All of the following explain the above except

   A. Availability of multiple routes of administration for haloperidol
   B. Availability of guided dosing strategies for haloperidol in delirium
   C. Lack of significant anticholinergic effect
   D. Lack of significant sedating properties
   E. Lack of significant hypotensive effect

42. Which of the following over-the-counter prescriptions used to enhance cognition is associated with coagulation dysfunction as a side-effect?

   A. Vitamin E
   B. Gingko biloba
   C. Oestrogen
   D. Selegiline
   E. Fish oils

43. In elderly people with failing eyesight Charles Bonnet syndrome is not uncommon. Which of the following features if present support the diagnosis?

   A. Auditory hallucinations
   B. Poor attention span
   C. Clear consciousness
   D. Generalized seizures
   E. Parkinsonian tremors

44. Senile self-neglect with significant reclusiveness in elderly people is called Diogenes syndrome. Which of the following is false with respect to this condition?

   A. Equal sex distribution
   B. Cannot be diagnosed in the absence of cognitive impairment
   C. Medical contact is often initiated by neighbours
   D. Associated with high degree of mortality
   E. Higher rates of personality disorders

45. The prevalence of potentially reversible dementia among all cases diagnosed with dementia is estimated to be around

   A. <1%
   B. <2%
   C. <5%
   D. <10%
   E. <20%

46. **Which of the following is true with regard to alcohol use disorders in elderly people?**
    A. The prevalence rates have been overestimated
    B. The safe weekly limit for an elderly man is 21 units
    C. The most common clinical presentation is symptoms of intoxication
    D. Lifetime alcohol consumption is an important indicator of alcohol use
    E. The CAGE questionnaire is not useful as a screening tool

47. **The most common perpetrators of elder abuse in private UK households are**
    A. Spouses
    B. Sons
    C. Care workers
    D. Siblings
    E. Neighbours

48. **All of the following are associated with a higher risk of elder abuse except**
    A. Diagnosis of dementia in the victim
    B. Perpetrator and victim living separately
    C. Social isolation of the victim
    D. Psychiatric diagnosis in the perpetrator
    E. Perpetrator being financially dependent on the victim

49. **Which of the following drugs has the least evidence in the form of randomized controlled trials (RCTs) for the management of behavioural and psychological symptoms of dementia?**
    A. Olanzapine
    B. Risperidone
    C. Haloperidol
    D. Zolpidem
    E. Rivastigmine

50. **Cholinesterase inhibitors are unlikely to be useful in the management of**
    A. Lewy body dementia
    B. Alzheimer's dementia
    C. Mixed dementia
    D. Frontotemporal dementia (FTD)
    E. Early-onset dementia of Alzheimer's type

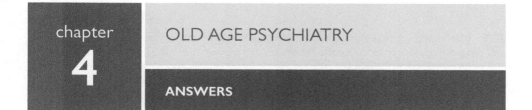

1. B. The process of ageing can be classified as primary ageing, which accounts for the relatively constant lifespan observed in a species, and secondary ageing, which explains much of the unpredictability among individual members of the species. The primary ageing process is most probably constitutional and is probably wired in the cellular machinery. This was demonstrated by Hayflick and colleagues, who showed that the maximum number of cell divisions that can occur in normal human cells in culture is approximately 40–60. Many functional capacities of the cells reduce as the cells approach the Hayflick limit. This 'Hayflick phenomenon' is under genetic control; it is not limited to laboratory culture methods. Pruning is a developmental phenomenon by which unnecessary synapses formed during brain development are removed. Apoptosis refers to programmed cell death.

Spar JE and Rue AL. *Clinical Manual of Geriatric Psychiatry.* American Psychiatric Publishing, 2006, p. 49.

2. D. The Hachinski Ischaemic Score is an easy-to-use clinical tool that aids in the bedside differentiation of Alzheimer's dementia from vascular dementia. It has been validated in patients with pathologically confirmed dementia. A cut-off score ≤4 supports a diagnosis of Alzheimer's dementia while a score ≥7 favours vascular dementia. These cut-off values have a sensitivity of 89% and a specificity of 89%. Abrupt onset, fluctuating course, history of stroke, presence of focal neurological symptoms and signs strongly favour a diagnosis of vascular dementia. Other supporting features for a diagnosis of vascular dementia include stepwise deterioration, presence of nocturnal confusion, absence of changes in personality, presence of emotional incontinence, depression and a history of hypertension.

Moroney JT. Meta-analysis of the Hachinski Ischaemic Score in pathologically verified dementias. *Neurology* 1997; **49**: 1096–1105.

3. A. In dementia complex ADL that require use of tools and equipment (instrumental ADLs) are affected earlier than basic ADL. Although self-report ADL measures are rare, they do exist. For example, the ADL-Prevention Instrument (ADL-PI) has a self-rated version and an informant version. Self-ratings are found to be closer to research observer's ratings, while family members tend to under-rate the ADL. Data from self-report of functioning predicts mortality better than informant data. The Barthel Index consists of 10 items that measure a person's ADL and mobility. It can be used to determine a baseline level of functioning and also to monitor changes in ADL over time. It is rated by carers or professionals. Currently, functional capacity measures are being used increasingly in pharmacological trials of patients with dementias as primary outcome measures. ADL scales are not gender biased and are commonly used in both sexes.

Massoud F. The role of functional assessment as an outcome measure in antidementia treatment. *Can J Neurol Sci* 2007; 34 Suppl 1: S47–51.

4. D. Huntington's disease is inherited in an autosomal dominant fashion. It is a neurodegenerative disorder related to expansion of a trinucleotide repeat sequence in the short arm of chromosome 4. Clinical features include a triad of choreic movements, cognitive decline, and psychiatric syndromes starting in the fourth to fifth decade. Psychiatric presentation is usually variable and can precede motor and cognitive changes. Most common psychiatric problems include change in personality (impulsive, disinhibited, and dissocial) and depression. Paranoid schizophrenia-like symptoms occur in 6–25% of cases. Such schizophrenia-like presentation is very rare in other conditions listed.

Correa B, Xavier M, and Guimaraes J. Association of Huntington's disease and schizophrenia-like psychosis in a Huntington's disease pedigree. *Clinical Practice and Epidemiology in Mental Health* 2006; **2**: 1.

5. D. Body composition changes with advancing age resulting in alterations in the way drugs are metabolized and circulated. Muscle mass and body water decline by as much as 25% by age 70 while the body lipid content increases. Body fat constitutes >40% of body weight in elderly women and >30% in elderly men. As a result, elderly people have a larger volume of distribution and longer half-life of lipophilic drugs. Lipid-soluble drugs such as diazepam have greater volume of distribution and half-life with slower clearance in elderly individuals.

Ginsberg G, Hattis D, Russ A, and Sonawane B. Pharmacokinetic and pharmacodynamic factors that can affect sensitivity to neurotoxic sequelae in elderly individuals. *Environmental Health Perspectives* 2005; **113**: 1243–1249.

6. A. The Neuropsychiatric inventory (NPI) can be used to measure behavioural and psychological features of dementia in elderly people. It was created by Cummings *et al.* It evaluates 10–12 neuropsychiatric disturbances common to dementia using frequency, severity and the carer's distress as indices. The Bristol scale is used to measure activities of daily living; the Cornell depression scale is used to assess depression in demented patients. The abbreviated mental test is a quick and easily administered test that is used as a screening tool for dementia.

Kaufer DI, Cummings JL, Ketchel P, *et al.* Validation of the NPI-Q, a brief clinical form of the Neuropsychiatric Inventory. *Journal of Neuropsychiatry and Clinical Neurosciences* 2000; **12**: 233–9.

7. C. The ADAS-Cog is used as the *de facto* standard primary outcome neuropsychological measure for dementia trials. It measures several cognitive domains, including memory, language, and praxis with total scores ranging from 0 to 70. A four-point change on the ADAS-Cog at 6 months after starting antidementia drugs has been used as an arbitrary cut-off point indicating a clinically important difference. This pharmaceutical cut-off on ADAS-Cog must be interpreted in the context of overall response when it is translated to clinical practice. MMSE is not as sensitive to change as ADAS-Cog; hence, it is rarely used as a primary outcome measure in dementia trials. An MRI brain scan currently has no role in monitoring treatment response.

Rockwood K, Fay S, Gorman M, *et al.* The clinical meaningfulness of ADAS-Cog changes in Alzheimer's disease patients treated with donepezil in an open-label trial. *BMC Neurology* 2007; **7**: 26.

8. B.   Alzheimer's dementia is associated with an annual decline on the MMSE of 3–4 points. Similarly using the ADAS-Cog scale, the natural disease progression averages a 7-point decline per year. But the average change on ADAS-Cog when using antidementia drugs is about 2.7 points. Thus cholinesterase inhibitors are considered to delay this progression by 6 months on average. MMSE is a reasonable tool for monitoring disease progression in a clinical setting, but the occurrence of functional impairment is more likely to be relevant to the patient and their carers than MMSE scores. Performance in instrumental activities of daily living such as telephone use, taking own medication, handling finances, and transport correlates well with cognitive impairment.

Woodford HJ and George J. Cognitive assessment in the elderly: a review of clinical methods. *QJM* 2007; **100**: 469–484.

9. A.   Generally, a high level of suspicion is needed to detect hyponatraemia in a depressed patient who does not undergo regular blood tests for electrolytes. The symptoms of hyponatraemia overlap with those of depression, making it hard to diagnose. Hyponatraemia due to selective serotonin reuptake inhibitors (SSRIs) or other antidepressant use is often linked to the syndrome of inappropriate antidiuretic hormone (SIADH) secretion. Increased age, female gender and co-prescription of diuretics are notable risk factors. Symptoms usually occur when the blood serum level falls below 130 mmol/L. These include lethargy, fatigue, muscle cramps, and headaches.

Baldwin R and Wild R. Management of depression in later life. *Advances in Psychiatric Treatment* 2004; **10**: 131–139.

10. E.   Plaques seen in the brain of patients with Alzheimer's dementia are insoluble extracellular deposits composed mainly of Aβ peptides. These Aβ peptides are derived from a transmembrane protein called B-amyloid precursor protein (APP) through proteolytic processing. APP is generally cleaved by β-secretase or α-secretase enzymes followed by γ-secretase. Aβ peptides are generated when APP is cleaved by β-secretase followed by γ-secretase. This pathway is amyloidogenic and forms the major metabolic pathway of APP in brain tissue; the non-amyloidogenic α-secretase pathway is the major pathway in other tissues. Presenilins are necessary for proteolytic activity of γ–secretase. PS/ γ-secretase complex is widely considered as a potential target for developing therapies against Alzheimer's disease.

Selkoe DJ. Presenilin, Notch, and the genesis and treatment of Alzheimer's disease. *Proceedings of the National Academy of Sciences USA* 2001; **98**: 11039–11041.

11. E.   DCM is an observational tool designed to evaluate the quality of care and well-being of people with dementia in formal care settings. It was designed by Kitwood in 1992. DCM is based on the social–psychological theory of dementia care, which states that much of the decline in patients with dementia is a direct consequence of the social and environmental situation experienced. Better social care may result in less suffering than would otherwise be expected from their neurological state. The Washington University CDR is a global scale developed to clinically denote the presence of Alzheimer's dementia and stage its clinical severity using semi-structured interviews with the patient and informants. The Burden Interview and Caregiver Burden Scale are used to measure the degree of caregiver strain.

Beavis D, Simpson S, and Graham I. A literature review of dementia care mapping: methodological considerations and efficacy. *Journal of Psychiatric and Mental Health Nursing* 2002; **9**: 725–736.

12. E. An array of various terms has been used to describe age-associated cognitive impairment not amounting to dementia. The most popular term is MCI, of which several types have been described of late. The amnestic MCI refers to the original description of MCI. Diagnosis of MCI requires the presence of memory complaint (preferably corroborated by an informant), objective memory impairment for age, preserved general cognitive function, normal functional activities, and no dementia. The presence or absence of family history of dementia is not a criterion used to describe MCI.

Chong MS, and Sahadevan S. Preclinical Alzheimer's disease: diagnosis and prediction of progression. *Lancet Neurology* 2005; **4**: 576–579.

13. D. The Lund–Manchester criteria are used in the diagnosis of frontotemporal dementia. The criteria were initially developed in 1994 and were later updated in 1998. The following core components are required for a diagnosis:

1. insidious onset and gradual progression
2. early decline in social interpersonal conduct
3. early impairment in regulation of personal conduct
4. early emotional blunting
5. early loss of insight

Other supportive diagnostic features include:

A. Behavioural disorder (decline in personal hygiene, mental rigidity and inflexibility, distractibility and impersistence, hyperorality and dietary change, utilization behaviour)
B. Speech and language disturbances (altered speech output, stereotypy of speech, echolalia, perseveration, mutism)
C Physical signs (primitive reflexes, incontinence, akinesia, rigidity, tremor)
D. Abnormal investigations (neuropsychological evidence of impaired frontal lobe function, normal conventional EEG despite clinically evident dementia and predominant frontal and/or anterior temporal abnormality in neuroimaging)

Gelder MG, et al., eds. *Shorter Oxford Textbook of Psychiatry*, 5th edn. Oxford University Press, 2006, p. 341.

14. B. Visual hallucinations dominate the clinical picture of dementia with Lewy bodies (DLB) in many patients. Visual hallucinations have a tendency to persist despite treatment in many patients. In phenomenological quality, the hallucinations of DLB are similar to those reported in Parkinson's disease dementia: they are vivid, colourful, three-dimensional, and generally mute images of animate objects. Visual hallucinations are associated with greater deficits in cortical acetylcholine and predict better response to cholinesterase inhibitors

McKeith I, Mintzer J, Aarsland D, et al. Dementia with Lewy bodies. *Lancet Neurology* 2004; **3**: 19–28.

15. C. It is reported that 25–50% of patients with DLB have extrapyramidal signs at the time of diagnosis, and another 25% develop extrapyramidal signs during the natural course of DLB. A quarter of all DLB patients have no extrapyramidal signs at all until death. So parkinsonism is not necessary for clinical diagnosis of DLB. Often a diagnosis of DLB is missed as clinicians look for extrapyramidal signs or suspect cerebrovascular disease. The pattern of extrapyramidal signs in DLB shows greater postural/gait instability and facial impassivity but less tremor. This pattern of parkinsonism is over-represented in both DLB and demented patients with Parkinson's disease. But non-demented Parkinson's disease patients show equal distribution of a tremor-dominant pattern and postural/gait instability pattern. It is possible that the tremor-related pattern is more dopamine-dependent dysfunction whereas postural/gait problems are more non-dopaminergic.

McKeith I, Mintzer J, Aarsland D, et al. Dementia with Lewy bodies. *Lancet Neurology* 2004; **3**: 19–28.

16. B. Multiple factors have been examined in an attempt to predict the treatment response in elderly depressed patients. A prospective study examining neurological and neuropsychological factors showed that a combination of extrapyramidal signs, pyramidal tract signs, and impairment of motor hand sequencing strongly predicted resistance to 12 weeks of antidepressant monotherapy, with 89% sensitivity and 95% specificity. Microstructural white matter abnormalities may also perpetuate depressive symptoms in older adults by disrupting connectivity with cortico-striato-limbic networks, which form the basis of mood regulation. Lower fractional anisotropy in this network predicted poorer treatment response in geriatric depression. Although enlarged cerebral ventricles have been reported in some studies, this is not examined as a predictor of treatment response. Earlier age of onset and somatic symptoms suggest better response to initial antidepressant treatment.

Simpson S, *et al.* Is subcortical disease associated with a poor response to antidepressants? Neurological, neuropsychological and neuroradiological findings in late-life depression. *Psychological Medicine* 1998; **28**: 1015–1026.

Alexopoulos GS and Murphy CF, Gunning-Dixon FM, *et al.* Microstructural white matter abnormalities and remission of geriatric depression. *American Journal of Psychiatry* 2008; **165**: 238–244.

17. C. Executive dysfunction predicts a poor or delayed response to antidepressant therapy and also a greater risk of relapse after discontinuing treatment. None of the other core symptoms of depression has been shown to be strong predictors of later relapse.

Kroenke K. A 75-year-old man with depression. *Journal of the American Medical Association* 2002; **287**: 1568–1576.

18. D. Late-life depression often occurs in the context of medical health issues; it is two to three times more common in the medically ill elderly patient. The diagnosis 'depression due to a general medical condition' (more commonly, secondary depression) is used when depressed mood or anhedonia occur in patients already diagnosed with an illness that is clearly linked to depression as a physiological consequence. For example, nearly 25% of patients with myocardial infarction have a major depressive episode. Primary depression can exist alongside a general medical condition with no direct physiological relationship. In fact, such co-existing depression and a general medical condition is more common than depression secondary to medical problems. Depression may also exacerbate the outcome of medical illnesses. Although hypothyroidism is considered to cause depression traditionally, recent studies show that a TSH value of 10 μU/L or greater was found in only 0.7% of elderly patients with clinical depression. Thus the rate of subclinical hypothyroidism in an elderly depressed group may be similar to that of the elderly population in general.

Kroenke K. A 75-year-old man with depression. *Journal of the American Medical Association* 2002; **287**: 1568–1576.

19. E. The term late-onset schizophrenia is applied to patients whose first symptom of schizophrenia-like psychosis begins after the age of 40. For patients whose symptoms begin after the age of 60, the term very-late-onset schizophrenia-like psychosis (VLOSLP) is used. Paranoid delusions are the most common symptoms in late-onset schizophrenia, followed by auditory hallucinations. Partition delusions are often noted in late/very late-onset schizophrenia where the patient typically believes that people, objects, or radiation can pass through what would normally constitute a barrier to such passage. Negative symptoms are conspicuously absent in most cases. In psychosis associated with Alzheimer's dementia, simple paranoid delusions are more common than hallucinations. In psychosis associated with Parkinson's disease, visual hallucinations are more common than delusions.

Mintzer J and Targum SD. Psychosis in elderly patients: classification and pharmacotherapy. *Journal of Geriatric Psychiatry and Neurology* 2003; **16**: 199–206.

Howard R, Castle D, O'Brien J, *et al*. Permeable walls, floors, ceilings and doors. Partition delusions in late paraphrenia. *International journal of geriatric psychiatry* 1992; **7**: 719–724.

20. A. Some individuals with abnormal grief reaction may be avoiding reminders of their grief, leading to unresolved emotions. Addressing these issues by encouragement may not be sufficient and a behavioural approach may be needed in some cases. The approach commonly used is known as guided mourning. This treats unresolved grief in a way similar to other forms of phobic avoidance by exposure to the avoided situation. Thus guided mourning involves intense reliving of avoided painful memories and feelings associated with bereavement. During treatment, patients are exposed to avoided painful memories or situations related to the loss of their loved one – both in imagination and in real life.

Clark A. Working with grieving adults. *Advances in Psychiatric Treatment* 2004; **10**: 164–170.

21. E. Elderly people with depression may have a relapse or recurrence of a depressive disorder from adulthood (early onset) or they might have fresh onset late-life depression. Late-onset major depression includes a large subgroup of patients with neurological problems. It is possible that milder, unnoticed episodes of depression with early-onset might be a risk factor for late-life depression by contributing to brain abnormalities. When compared with elderly individuals with early-onset major depression, patients with late-onset major depression have a less frequent family history of mood disorders, a higher prevalence of disorders of dementia, a larger impairment in neuropsychological tests, a higher rate of dementia development on follow-up, more neurosensory hearing impairment, a greater enlargement in lateral brain ventricles, and more white matter hyperintensities.

Alexopoulos GS. Depression in the elderly. *Lancet* 2005; **365**: 1961–1970.

22. C. A systematic review of studies looking at improvements in caregiver psychological health revealed that six or more sessions of individual behavioural management therapy had the highest quality of evidence. This intervention was effective for up to 32 months after intervention. There was some evidence supporting individual and group caregiver coping sessions to reduce depression among caregivers; the benefits may last up to 3 months. Educational interventions, group behavioural management sessions, fewer than six individual behavioural management sessions, and supportive therapy were not effective interventions for reducing a caregiver's symptoms.

Selwood A, Johnston K, Katona C, *et al*. Systematic review of the effect of psychological interventions on family caregivers of people with dementia. *Journal of Affective Disorders* 2007; **101**: 75–89.

23. A.　Reminiscence therapy uses materials such as old newspapers and household items to stimulate memories and enable people to share and value their experiences. The evidence base for this therapy in improving behavioural problems is limited. It may have a modest impact on mood symptoms. Validation therapy is based on Rogerian humanistic psychology; it encourages individual uniqueness and gives the opportunity to resolve conflicts by encouraging and validating the expression of feelings and emotions. Reality orientation therapy is based on the fact that patients with dementia function poorly secondary to impairment in orientating information (day, date, weather, time, and use of names) Hence reminders can improve functioning. Cognitive stimulation therapy is similar to reality orientation therapy but aims at improving information processing rather than factual knowledge to address problems in functioning in patients with dementia. Snoezelen therapy is also called multisensory stimulation. It is grounded on the supposition that neuropsychiatric symptoms may result from periods of sensory deprivation. It combines relaxation and exploration of sensory stimuli (e.g. lights, sounds, and tactile sensations).

Livingston G, Johnston K, Katona C, et al. Systematic review of psychological approaches to the management of neuropsychiatric symptoms of dementia. American Journal of Psychiatry 2005; **162**: 1996–2021.

24. D.　Psychosis is a prominent non-cognitive symptom seen in Alzheimer's dementia. The prevalence of psychosis in patients with Alzheimer's dementia has been estimated at 30–50%. Psychotic symptoms are seen in 0.2–4.7% of the elderly population in the community. In nursing homes the prevalence rates are very high – 10–60%. Dementia accounts for the highest number of psychotic symptoms diagnosed among elderly people. Prospective studies have shown that 36.7% of patients with psychotic symptoms may have dementia, most likely of Alzheimer's type.

Holroyd S and Laurie S. Correlates of psychotic symptoms among elderly outpatients. International Journal of Geriatric Psychiatry 1999; **14**: 379–384.

25. A.　Bowlby and Parkes proposed a stage theory of grief for adjustment to bereavement that included four stages: shock–numbness, yearning–searching, disorganization–despair, and reorganization. This was adapted by Kubler-Ross, who described a five-stage response of terminally ill patients to impending death: **d**enial–dissociation–isolation, **a**nger, **b**argaining, **d**epression, and **a**cceptance (mnemonic: DABDA). A longitudinal cohort study (Yale Bereavement Study) has established that in terms of absolute frequency, disbelief was not the initial grief indicator as proposed by the original grief theory. The study found that most people endorsed acceptance as initial reaction even in the initial month after loss in cases of natural deaths. In contrast, family members of those who had a traumatic death and individuals with complicated grief disorder had significantly lower levels of acceptance. It was also noted that prognostic awareness of a patient's terminal illness for more than 6 months before death may promote acceptance of the death.

Maciejewski PK, Zhang B, Block SD, and Prigerson HG. An empirical examination of the stage theory of grief. Journal of the American Medical Association 2007; **297**: 716–723.

26. E. The presence of hippocampal atrophy in patients with amnestic MCI may predict the onset of later dementia. The risk of conversion to dementia is four times higher in 5 years when hippocampal atrophy is present. It is generally accepted that the closer one's cognitive ability, brain imaging, and genetic susceptibility are to AD, the more likely is the progression to dementia from MCI. Other factors predicting conversion include older age, greater severity of baseline cognitive deficits, especially impaired episodic recall and hypoperfusion of multiple brain regions in neuroimaging studies. It is also noted that multidomain amnestic MCI has a higher conversion rate than pure amnestic MCI. This conversion is more pronounced if the cognitive complaints are accompanied by carers' reports of impaired daily function. Sensory impairment has no role in such predictions.

DeCarli C. Mild cognitive impairment: prevalence, prognosis, aetiology, and treatment. *Lancet Neurology* 2003; **2**: 15–21.

27. A. It is very difficult to conclusively decide on epidemiological facts of mild cognitive impairment due to the variations in diagnostic terms and inclusion criteria used in epidemiological research. A prevalence between 3% and 19% has been reported in elderly people. The age-specific prevalence of MCI is greater than that of dementia. MCI is about four times more common than dementia when based on community assessment of non-institutionalized individuals. An incidence of 8–58 per 1000 per year and a risk of developing dementia of 11–33% over 2 years have been quoted. The progression of amnestic MCI to dementia has been examined in various clinical populations. Generally a yearly incidence of dementia of 10–15% has been quoted for those with MCI attending memory clinics (compare this with general rates of 1–2% in elderly people). Community-based studies show slightly lower rates of conversion closer to 5–10% per year. A significant number of those with amnestic MCI actually improve their cognitive performance during follow up. Up to 44% of patients with mild cognitive impairment are estimated to return to normal a year later.

Gauthier S, Reisberg B, Zaudig M, *et al*. Mild cognitive impairment. *Lancet* 2006; **367**: 1262–1270.

28. C. It is important to note that AD by itself is not a fatal disease. The median survival time following a diagnosis of AD depends strongly on the patient's age at diagnosis. The older the age at diagnosis, the higher the chances of death. For example, some studies have shown a difference in median survival time of around 5 years between those diagnosed with dementia at the age of 65 and those diagnosed at the age of 90. The median survival from initial diagnosis is higher for men than women in some studies but this is not consistently shown. The presence of frontal lobe release signs, extrapyramidal signs, and gait disturbance, history of falls, congestive heart failure, ischaemic heart disease, and diabetes at baseline may predict shorter survival. Based on numerous longitudinal studies, a median survival of 5–8 years has been estimated. A multicentre prospective population-based cohort study in England and Wales with 14 years' follow-up reported median survival after the estimated onset of dementia as 4.6 years for women and 4.1 years for men. There was a difference of nearly 7 years in survival between the younger old and the oldest people with dementia: 10.7 years for ages 65–69 vs. 3.8 years for ages ≥90. Significant factors that predicted mortality in the presence of dementia during the follow-up included sex, age of onset, and disability before the onset. Type of accommodation, marital status, and self-reported health were not associated with survival.

Gelder MG *et al*., eds. *Shorter Oxford Textbook of Psychiatry*, 5th edn. Oxford University Press, 2006, p. 336.
Larson EB, Shadlen M-F, Wang L, *et al*. Survival after Initial Diagnosis of Alzheimer Disease. *Annals of Internal Medicine* 2004; **140**: 501–509.
Xie J, Brayne C, and Matthews FE *et al*. Survival times in people with dementia: analysis from population based cohort study with 14 year follow up. *British Medical Journal* 2008; **10**: 1136.

29. D.   Braak's staging system has been used to grade pathologically the various degrees of dementia severity. It is based on the appearance of neurofibrillary tangles in brain. These tangles commence the transentorhinal and entorhinal cortex spreading to the hippocampus, and then extend across the remaining limbic system before involving other cortical regions, followed by the primary motor and somatosensory cortices, and finally the occipital cortex. This progression is the basis of the Braak's staging. A decline in memory test performance and mental state of the demented patient correlate with the pathological progression through the neocortical Braak stages.

Gelder MG, *et al.*, eds. *Shorter Oxford Textbook of Psychiatry*, 5th edn. Oxford University Press, 2006, p. 337.

30. A.   The term Binswanger's disease refers to a type of subcortical vascular dementia caused by widespread, microscopic atherosclerotic vascular damage to the deep white matter in the brain. As a result patients may have frontal *executive dysfunction,* short-term memory loss, and behavioural changes. The most characteristic feature is said to be the reduction of processing speed. An MRI scan of the brain can reveal the characteristic brain lesions essential for diagnosis. Single large infarcts or multiple cortical infarcts give rise to vascular dementia. Periventricular white matter lesions are non-specific and are commonly seen in Alzheimer's dementia, extreme ageing with vascular risk factors, and also in patients with frank vascular dementia.

Nagata K, Saito H, Ueno T, *et al.* Clinical diagnosis of vascular dementia. *Journal of the Neurological Sciences* 2007; **257**: 44–48.

31. B.   An actual predicted risk of developing Alzheimer's disease in first-degree relatives of probands with Alzheimer's disease is 15–19%, compared with 5% in controls. Thus, the risk to first-degree relatives of patients with Alzheimer's disease who developed the disorder at any time up to the age of 85 years is increased to 3–4 times relative to the risk in controls. This would seem to translate to a risk of developing Alzheimer's disease of between one in five and one in six.

Liddell, *et al.* Genetic risk of Alzheimer's disease: advising relatives. *The British Journal of Psychiatry* 2001; **178**: 7–11.

32. C.   The core neuropathology of CJD is characterized by spongiform change, neuronal loss, astrocytosis, and amyloid plaque formation. The amyloid plaques in CJD are generally made of insoluble prion proteins. In addition, abnormal neuritic dendrites with white matter necrosis and beta protein amyloid angiopathy may also be seen.

Tetsuyuki KJT, Takatoshi T, Takeshita I, *et al.* Amyloid plaques in Creutzfeldt-Jakob disease stain with prion protein antibodies. *Annals of Neurology* 1986; **20**: 204–208.

33. B.   vCJD causes rapidly progressive dementia, often leading to death in relatively young patients. Symmetrical hyperintensity in the posterior nuclei of the thalamus, called the pulvinar sign, is seen on brain MRI images of most patients with vCJD. This is described as a specific, non-invasive, and highly accurate diagnostic sign of vCJD; FLAIR (fluid-attenuated inversion recovery) sequences are more sensitive than T1 weighted, T2 weighted or proton density MRI. The pulvinar sign is reported to have a sensitivity of 78% and specificity of 100%. The pulvinar sign has been so far demonstrated only in symptomatic patients; its validity as a screening test in presymptomatic patients is unclear.

Macfarlane RG, Wroe SJ, Collinge J, *et al.* Neuroimaging findings in human prion disease. *Journal of Neurology, Neurosurgery, and Psychiatry* 2007; **78**: 664–670.

34. A. Phobic disorders are the most common neurotic conditions noted in epidemiological studies of elderly people. Despite great variations in the reported rates of all neurotic disorders in elderly people, the overall prevalence of neurotic disorders is thought to vary between 2.5% and 14.2% of the population aged 65 years or older. The reported prevalence of phobic disorders varies enormously from 1.4% to 25.6% in various studies due to differences in the instruments used, and variable application of hierarchical case ascertainment rules when dealing with agoraphobia. More recently, a longitudinal population study from Europe reported current prevalence rates of 14.2% for anxiety disorders as a whole, 10.7% for phobia, 4.6% for generalized anxiety disorder, 3% for major depression, and 1.7% for psychosis in elderly people.

Ritchie K, Artero S, Beluche I, et al. Prevalence of DSM-IV psychiatric disorder in the French elderly population. *British Journal of Psychiatry* 2004; **184**: 147–152.

Bryant C, Jackson H, and Ames D. The prevalence of anxiety in older adults: Methodological issues and a review of the literature. *Journal of Affective Disorders* 2008; **109**: 233–250.

35. A. Older patients who commit suicide are more likely to suffer from depressive illness but are less likely to be known to mental health services or to have been treated for depression than younger adults who kill themselves. It is also known that older people are more likely to enter into suicide pacts. In older people, male suicide rates are higher than female suicides. It is generally accepted that the conversion rate of suicidal thoughts to acts is higher in older patients.

Murray R, Kendler K, et al., eds. *Essential Psychiatry*, 4th edn. Cambridge University Press, 2008, p. 374.

36. D. Testamentary capacity refers to the competence for drafting and signing a will. In English law, this is based on case *Banks* v *Goodfellow* in 1870. The capacity to draw a will requires

1. understanding the nature of the act of drawing a will and its effects
2. understanding the extent of the property being disposed
3. understanding the nature and extent of the claims of those who are included or excluded in the will
4. absence of mental disorder that can affect the previous (1–3) competencies
5. absence of undue influence (duress) by third parties.

Hence a mentally ill individual can have full testamentary capacity if his/her mental illness does not directly influence his/her understanding of the process, the extent of his/her estate, or the nature of claims that could be made to his/her estate.

Murray B and Jacoby R. The interface between old age psychiatry and the law. *Advances in Psychiatric Treatment* 2002; **8**: 271–278.

37. D. Late-life mania is often different from earlier onset mania. There is a prominent mixture of depressive symptoms in late-life mania; in addition, those with late-onset mania are more likely to have had a depressed phase during their first admission. Occasionally, manic symptoms in late life may herald the onset of frontal-type dementia. It is also shown that men may have higher rates of mania in late-life than women – one series reported a difference of 60% in men to 10% in women. A significant association with cerebral organic disease has been demonstrated, leading to the term secondary mania in cases with organic aetiology. A higher tendency to find vascular lesions in neuroimaging studies of older manic patients has been described. Similar to geriatric depression, late-life mania is also said to have less genetic contribution to aetiology than younger adults with mania.

Murray R, Kendler K, et al., eds. *Essential Psychiatry*, 4th edn. Cambridge University Press, 2008, p. 369.

38. D. Tacrine, donepezil, and galantamine selectively inhibit acetylcholinesterase. In addition galantamine also improves cholinergic neurotransmission by acting as an allosteric ligand at nicotinic acetylcholine receptors to increase presynaptic acetylcholine release and postsynaptic neurotransmission. Rivastigmine inhibits butyrylcholinesterase in addition to its inhibition of acetylcholinesterase. Butyrylcholinesterase forms around 10% of the total cholinesterase in normal human brains and it is mainly associated with glial cells. With the progression of dementia, it is noted that acetylcholinesterase activity decreases while butyrylcholinesterase activity stabilizes or even increases in relation to glial proliferation. This may lead to changes in the ratio of acetylcholinesterase to butyrylcholinesterase. To date, a significant difference in the clinical efficacy of rivastigmine compared with donepezil or galantamine in advanced dementia has not been demonstrated

Scarpini E, Schelterns P, and Feldman H. Treatment of Alzheimer's disease; current status and new perspectives. *Lancet Neurology* 2003; **2**: 539–547.

39. C. Memantine is a non-competitive NMDA antagonist that prevents excess calcium from entering the neurons leading to a neuroprotective effect. It is completely absorbed from the gastrointestinal tract with a bioavailability of 100%. Memantine exhibits linear (first order) pharmacokinetics over the entire dosage range of 10–40 mg/day. It rapidly passes the blood–brain barrier within 30 minutes of absorption. Forty-five per cent of the drug binds to plasma proteins. It is metabolized by glucuronidation, hydroxylation, and N-oxidation. Seventy-five to 90% of the drug is eliminated via the urine, with 10–25% of the drug eliminated in the bile and faeces. The elimination half-life is about 60–80 hours. Excessively alkaline urine can decrease the excretion.

Robinson DM, Keating GM. Memantine: a review of its use in Alzheimer's disease. *Drugs* 2006; **66**: 1515–1534.

40. C. Head-to-head comparisons of antidementia drugs show similar effects on measures of cognition and behaviour for rivastigmine, galantamine, and donepezil. But the analysis of withdrawals before the end of the study period showed significant differences between donepezil and other medications in the group – especially rivastigmine. Similarly, a meta-analysis that compared the effect of galantamine, rivastigmine, and donepezil on safety (drop-outs due to adverse events) and selected cognitive outcomes showed a comparable benefit on ADAS-Cog scores compared with placebo for all three drugs; a dose-related effect was observed for donepezil and rivastigmine but not galantamine. There was evidence for increased drop-out rates with both galantamine and rivastigmine compared with donepezil.

Tyrer P and Silk K., eds. *Cambridge Textbook of Effective Treatments in Psychiatry.* Cambridge University Press, 2008, p 224.

41. B. Many practice guidelines for the treatment of patients with delirium support the use of antipsychotics as the drugs of choice in delirium. Haloperidol is the most frequently used due to the different available routes of administration, a lack of anticholinergic side-effects, few active metabolites, and the low likelihood of causing adverse effects such as sedation and hypotension, which can be difficult to manage in an acute confusional state. But as QT prolongation is a possible side-effect, it is advisable to have a baseline ECG before such use is attempted in high-risk patients. These recommendations do not have much evidence base but are largely driven by retrospective chart surveys; hence, there is a dearth of data on dosage guidance. It is suggested that haloperidol is given at half the adult dose in elderly people.

Tyrer P and Silk K., eds. *Cambridge Textbook of Effective Treatments in Psychiatry.* Cambridge University Press, 2008, p 181.

42. B. Gingko biloba extract is widely used as a herbal preparation for dementia and other cognitive difficulties. Gingko has a significant effect on prostaglandin metabolism and it antagonizes the platelet aggregating factor. As a result platelet function may be compromised especially when other anticoagulants like warfarin are co-administered. Many cases of internal bleeding and postoperative bleeding have been attributed to Gingko. Monitoring bleeding time may be an option in high-risk patients, but this is only a crude measure of platelet dysfunction.

Fong KCS and Kinnear PE. Retrobulbar haemorrhage associated with chronic Gingko biloba ingestion. *Postgraduate Medical Journal* 2003; **79**: 531–532.

43. C. Charles Bonnet syndrome is a common cause of complex visual hallucination in elderly people. 10% to 15% of visually impaired elderly patients may have this syndrome. The eponym comes from the Swiss naturalist and philosopher Charles Bonnet, who reported the hallucinations of his 89-year-old grandfather, who was blind with cataracts but saw multiple animated objects. Core features of Charles Bonnet syndrome include the occurrence of recurrent well-formed, vivid, elaborate, and often stereotyped visual hallucinations in a partially sighted person. The patient usually retains insight into the unreal nature of the images. It is important to consider other differential diagnoses, such as Lewy body dementia, psychosis, delirium, neurological illness, and intoxication.

Manford M and Andermann F. Complex visual hallucinations. Clinical and neurobiological insights. *Brain* 1998; **121**: 1819–40.

44. B. Patients with so-called Diogenes syndrome are characterized by aloofness and breakdown of self-care to a severe extent; in some cases they may pose an environmental health hazard. Many of them are resistant to intervention from any agency, including relatives. Men and women are equally affected, but the condition is rare. An annual incidence of 0.5 per 1000 of the population aged over 60 years is reported. Diogenes syndrome is not a diagnostic category and patients form a heterogeneous group with respect to diagnoses. Some of them may have personality disorders, some have dementia while some are diagnosed with late-onset schizophrenia. Overall mortality is high for such patients.

Murray R, Kendler K, *et al.*, eds. *Essential Psychiatry*, 4th edn. Cambridge University Press, 2008, p. 374–75.

45. D. Traditionally an optimistically high rate of 10–20% of diagnosed dementia was thought to be due to reversible causes. A systematic review and meta-analysis of evidence in this regard shows a much lower rate of dementia due to potentially reversible causes to be 9% and actual (partial or full) reversal takes place in only 0.6%. Potentially reversible causes tend to be seen more in relatively young patients or in those with more recent onset of symptoms. It is not clear if an improvement in diagnostic practices in primary care has contributed to a lower proportion of patients with reversible dementia being referred. Depression being wrongly diagnosed as dementia forms the major proportion of reversible dementia; metabolic and endocrine issues such as hypothyroidism, vitamin B12 deficiency are other common causes. Subdural haematoma, cerebral tumours, and normal pressure hydrocephalus can cause potentially reversible dementias, although the degree of reversibility is controversial.

Clarfield AM. The decreasing prevalence of reversible dementias: an updated meta-analysis. *Archives of Internal Medicine* 2003; **163**: 2219–2229.

46. D.   The prevalence of alcohol use disorders in elderly people is generally lower than in younger adults, but it is generally accepted that the rates are underestimated because of underdetection and misdiagnosis. It is known that elicitation and documentation of alcohol misuse in the medical records of the elderly people is poor. In addition, elderly people are less likely to spontaneously disclose alcohol use. Even in those identified with alcohol misuse, referral to a specialist team is very low, probably due to a degree of existing therapeutic nihilism (the belief that the illness is incurable) among health workers. Alcohol problems often present atypically in elderly people – falls, confusion, and depression are common presentations. It is also often masked by poor physical health . Furthermore, weekly limits of sensible drinking for adults, i.e. 21 units for men and 14 units for women, may not apply to elderly people. This is due to age-related changes in the pharmacokinetics of alcohol. In most countries, age-appropriate limits have not been established for elderly people. A history of lifetime alcohol consumption may be more important than current levels of drinking to ascertain the degree of alcohol use in elderly people. The CAGE questionnaire has relatively good sensitivity and specificity in older people, but, compared with younger adults, it works better in elderly people when supplemented by further questions.

O'Connell H, Chin A-V, Cunningham C, *et al.* Alcohol use disorders in elderly people-redefining an age old problem in old age. *British Medical Journal* 2003; **327**: 664–667.

47. A.   Fieldwork carried out in the UK by the National Centre for Social research showed that 2.6% (1 in 40) of people aged 66 and over living in private households had experienced abuse (from family, friends, or care workers) in the past year. Neglect is the predominant form of mistreatment, followed by financial, physical, and psychological abuse. The rates of sexual abuse were low. Partners (51%) and other family members (49%) were most commonly reported as the perpetrators of mistreatment compared with care workers (13%) or friends (5%).

O'Keeffe M, Hills A, Doyle M, *et al. UK Study of Abuse and Neglect of Older People: Prevalence survey report.* National Centre for Social Research, 2007.

48. B.   Various risk factors have been proposed from prospective analysis of elder abuse. Shared living situation is a major risk factor; older people living alone are at lowest risk. Having a 'poor social network' and subsequent social isolation significantly increases the risk of mistreatment. A diagnosis of dementia makes elderly people more vulnerable to mistreatment. The prevalence rates of elder abuse in samples of dementia caregivers is far higher than the elder abuse seen in the general community. Similarly, a higher rate of mental illness, such as depression or substance abuse, among caregivers increases the risk of elder abuse. It is also found that perpetrators of elder abuse tend to be financially dependent on the abused individual.

Lachs, MS and Pillemer, K. Elder abuse. *Lancet 2004;* **364**: 1263–1273.

49. D.   Evidence from RCT exists for the treatment of behavioural and psychological symptoms of dementia (BPSD) using atypical antipsychotics, such as olanzapine and risperidone, typical antipsychotics, such as haloperidol, and cholinesterase inhibitors. In addition, RCT evidence exists for use of antidepressants for depressive symptoms in dementia. RCTs suggest an approximate doubling in the risk of cerebrovascular accidents in patients receiving risperidone, olanzapine, or quetiapine. Zolpidem has a weak evidence base for use in BPSD; it may help insomnia in elderly patients with dementia.

Tyrer P and Silk K., eds. *Cambridge Textbook of Effective Treatments in Psychiatry.* Cambridge University Press, 2008, p 191.

50. D.   Cholinesterase inhibitors have been shown to be useful in the treatment of senile dementia of Alzheimer's type, mixed Alzheimer's and vascular dementia, Lewy body dementia, Parkinson's disease dementia, and young onset Alzheimer's-type dementia. Too date, there is no evidence of reasonable quality to recommend their use in FTD. Normal levels of cholinacetyltransferase have been demonstrated in patients with FTD compared with reduced levels seen in Alzheimer's disease; this might explain the lack of efficacy of cholinesterase inhibitors in FTD.

Gelder MG, *et al.*, eds. *Shorter Oxford Textbook of Psychiatry*, 5th edn. Oxford University Press, 2006, p. 511.

1. According to Jellinek's classification of alcoholism, which of the following types refers to a person who has developed physical and psychological dependence but still maintains the ability to abstain if necessary?
   A. Alpha
   B. Beta
   C. Gamma
   D. Delta
   E. Epsilon

2. Which of the following is NOT a criterion for alcohol dependence syndrome as described by Edwards and Gross?
   A. A subjective awareness of compulsion to drink
   B. Increased tolerance to alcohol
   C. Repeated withdrawal symptoms
   D. Relief or avoidance of withdrawal symptoms by further drinking
   E. Reduction in social obligations

3. Which of the following is NOT a diagnostic criterion for alcohol dependence according to DSM-IV?
   A. Strong desire or sense of compulsion to drink alcohol
   B. Tolerance
   C. Withdrawal
   D. Loss of normal social activities due to drinking
   E. Continued intake despite knowledge of the harmful effect

4. The mortality rate in a person being treated for alcohol withdrawal delirium is
   A. 0–1%
   B. 10–20%
   C. 20–30%
   D. 30–40%
   E. >50%

5. **What is the typical time period in which withdrawal delirium appears in an alcohol-dependent person who has stopped drinking?**
    A. Within 6 hours
    B. 6–12 hours
    C. 2–3 days
    D. After 7 days
    E. 2 weeks

6. **A patient who was found to be unconscious on the roadside was brought to the A&E. While transporting him, he had a seizure in the ambulance. Which of the following best points towards a diagnosis of generalized epilepsy rather than a seizure associated with alcohol-related complications?**
    A. Electrolyte disturbances
    B. Hypoglycaemia
    C. Occult subdural haematoma
    D. Presence of illicit substances in the drug screen
    E. Generalized spikes and waves on the inter-ictal EEG

7. **Which of the following is the treatment of choice for status epilepticus in a case of alcohol withdrawal?**
    A. Diazepam
    B. Chlordiazepoxide
    C. Lorazepam
    D. Carbamazepine
    E. Phenytoin

8. **Which of the following is a relative contraindication in a case of alcohol withdrawal delirium?**
    A. Diazepam
    B. Lorazepam
    C. Haloperidol
    D. Chlorpromazine
    E. Chlordiazepoxide

9. **Failure to diagnose and failure to institute adequate thiamine replacement therapy for Wernicke's encephalopathy is associated with a mortality of nearly**
    A. 5%
    B. 10%
    C. 20%
    D. 30%
    E. >50%

10. **If left untreated what percentage of people who develop Wernicke's encephalopathy goes on to develop a severe persistent amnestic syndrome (Korsakoff's dementia)?**

    A. 5%
    B. 10%
    C. 20%
    D. 40%
    E. 75%

11. **A severely malnourished patient is admitted to hospital for planned surgery. He develops alcohol withdrawal delirium. He has no signs of Wernicke's encephalopathy. Which of the following is the best strategy for thiamine replacement in this patient?**

    A. Oral thiamine 30 mg three times daily for 5 days
    B. Oral thiamine 50 mg three times daily for 5 days
    C. Intravenous thiamine 250 mg three times daily for 5 days
    D. Intramuscular thiamine 50 mg three times daily for 5 days
    E. Thiamine is not required as the patient has not developed Wernicke's encephalopathy

12. **Which of the following is not a risk factor for suicide in an alcohol-dependent individual?**

    A. Male gender
    B. Age less than 50 years
    C. Recent interpersonal loss event
    D. Poor social circumstances
    E. Polysubstance use

13. **Lifetime prevalence rates of alcohol use disorder is highest in**

    A. Bipolar disorder
    B. Schizophrenia
    C. Panic disorder
    D. Major depression
    E. Generalized anxiety disorder

14. **Psychosocial interventions available for alcohol dependence include motivational enhancement therapy (MET), cognitive behavioural therapy (CBT) and 12-step facilitation programmes (TSF). Which of the following is NOT correct with regard to these interventions?**

    A. Four sessions of MET were found to be equivalent to 12 sessions of CBT
    B. MET was more cost-effective than CBT
    C. High levels of anger at baseline predicted better outcomes with CBT than MET
    D. Participants in Alcoholics Anonymous (AA) responded better with TSF than MET
    E. 'Meaning-seeking' patients fared better on TSF than MET

15. **Which of the following clients are the most suitable for using brief interventions for alcohol use?**

    A. Problem drinkers attending primary care
    B. Prisoners with physical health problems due to alcohol use
    C. Moderate alcohol dependence
    D. Severe alcohol dependence
    E. Relapse prevention therapy following achievement of abstinence

16. **In the United Kingdom, one unit of alcohol is equivalent to which of the following?**

    A. 4 grams of pure alcohol
    B. 6 grams of pure alcohol
    C. 8 grams of pure alcohol
    D. 12 grams of pure alcohol
    E. 24 grams of pure alcohol

17. **Which of the following is incorrect with regard to the pharmacokinetics of alcohol?**

    A. Most alcohol is absorbed from the small intestine
    B. Pylorospasm can reduce the amount of absorption
    C. Women are less likely to get intoxicated than men for a given dose
    D. A fixed amount of alcohol gets metabolized in the liver irrespective of plasma concentration
    E. Absorption of alcohol is inhibited by the presence of food in the stomach

18. **Which of the following has been found to be the best screening method for hazardous drinking in primary care settings?**

    A. Alcohol Use Disorders Identification Test (AUDIT)
    B. CAGE questionnaire
    C. Mean corpuscular volume
    D. Gamma glutamyltransferase levels
    E. MAST

19. **Which of the following is true with regard to alcoholic blackouts?**

    A. They consist of discrete episodes of anterograde amnesia
    B. Loss of memory for the remote past is a characteristic feature
    C. Acute thiamine depletion is the causative factor
    D. Alcoholic blackouts are rare among binge drinkers
    E. Epileptiform activity is almost always noted in EEG during blackouts

20. **Which of the following is least likely to be a presenting physical feature of a child with foetal alcohol syndrome (FAS)?**

    A. Macrocephaly
    B. Learning disability
    C. Absent philtrum
    D. Syndactyly
    E. Atrial septal defect

21. **Mr White is an 80-year-old gentleman who has been taking diazepam at a dose of 20 mg at night for the past 3 years. During a trip to France to meet his nephew, he forgets to take his medication. Which of the following is NOT likely to be a seen if he experiences benzodiazepine withdrawal?**

   A. Delirium
   B. Anxiety
   C. Bursts of high-frequency activity on the EEG
   D. Insomnia
   E. Nightmares

22. **Polymorphisms of genes encoding which of the following enzymes/receptors confers protection from alcohol dependence in certain ethnic groups?**

   A. Aldehyde dehydrogenase (ALDH)
   B. Amino acid dehydrogenase
   C. GABA$_A$ receptor
   D. CYP3A4 enzyme
   E. HLA-DR2 protein

23. **Which of the following statements regarding alcohol use and comorbid depression is correct?**

   A. 10–20% of clients who use alcohol have at least one episode of depression in their lifetime
   B. Abstinence from alcohol does not lead to recovery from depression
   C. Women with alcohol problems have more comorbid depression than men
   D. Alcohol reduces the likelihood of successful completion of suicide among the depressed
   E. Risk of depression is independent of the amount of alcohol consumed daily

24. **Which of the following best describes the mechanism of action of Acamprosate?**

   A. GABA$_A$ partial agonism
   B. Blockade of ADH
   C. Competitive antagonism of ALDH
   D. Modulating opioid system to reduce craving
   E. Reducing post-synaptic glutamate neurotransmission at NMDA receptor

25. **Sam has been diagnosed with alcohol dependence. He has been started on disulfiram following a planned detoxification. You educate him about the effects and side-effects of the medication. Unfortunately, Sam decides to start drinking again after taking disulfiram for 3 weeks. How long should he wait after stopping disulfiram before he can be sure of having no unpleasant side-effects?**

   A. 1–2 hours
   B. 1–2 days
   C. 2–7 days
   D. 1–2 weeks
   E. 1–2 months

26. **Learning to walk in a straight line despite the motor impairment produced by alcohol intoxication is best explained by which of the following?**

    A. Pharmacodynamic tolerance
    B. Pharmacokinetic tolerance
    C. Behavioural tolerance
    D. Conditioned tolerance
    E. Reverse tolerance

27. **Which of the following is NOT a principle used during motivational interviewing of substance users?**

    A. Expressing empathy
    B. Helping the client to see discrepancies in their behaviours
    C. Avoiding argument
    D. Resisting resistance
    E. Supporting the patient's sense of self-efficacy

28. **Which of the following is NOT a risk factor for the development of alcohol hallucinosis?**

    A. Severe alcohol dependence
    B. Later age of onset of alcohol problems
    C. Binge drinking
    D. Higher rate of other substance use
    E. Family history of schizophrenia

29. **A decrease in which of the following subtypes of dopamine receptors makes an individual susceptible to relapse in a population with substance use?**

    A. D1
    B. D2
    C. D3
    D. D4
    E. D5

30. **Which of the following is NOT shown to be associated with an increase in the risk of development of alcohol abuse in elderly people?**

    A. Family history of alcohol use
    B. Presence of an organic mental disorder
    C. Having a drinking partner
    D. Grief
    E. Social isolation

31. **Mr Smith is diagnosed with alcohol dependence syndrome. He receives an educational session regarding the effects of drinking and the potential benefits of abstinence. He does not make any immediate change in his attitude or behaviour but is prepared to consider altering his drinking habits. Which of the following phases of Prochaska's transtheoretical model of change is he in?**

    A. Preparation
    B. Precontemplation
    C. Contemplation
    D. Action
    E. Maintenance

32 **Which of the following best describes the learning theory behind the efficacy of supervised disulfiram treatment?**

    A. Aversion theory
    B. Positive reinforcement
    C. Negative reinforcement
    D. Punishment theory
    E. Deterrence theory

33. **Which of the following is the most common intracranial complication of cocaine use?**

    A. Non-haemorrhagic infarct
    B. Transient ischaemic attack (TIA)
    C. Subarachnoid haemorrhage
    D. Intraventricular haemorrhage
    E. Intraparenchymal haemorrhage

34. **Chris and Ken are classmates at the local primary school. Chris's father has problems related to alcohol use, while Ken's parents are teetotal. How many times is Chris more likely to develop an alcohol-related problem in later life than Ken, assuming other psychosocial factors are comparable?**

    A. 2–3 times
    B. 4–10 times
    C. 10–20 times
    D. 20–40 times
    E. 100 times

35. **Which of the following is the most common lifetime comorbid diagnosis in a person with cocaine dependence?**

    A. Alcohol use disorder
    B. Depression
    C. Antisocial personality disorder
    D. Phobia
    E. Schizophrenia

36. **Which of the following is a factor that can increase the risk of benzodiazepine withdrawal in a clinical setting?**
    A. Gradual tapering of the prescribed drug
    B. Shorter duration of exposure
    C. Low level of psychopathology before initiation of benzodiazepine D treatment
    D. Low level of educational attainment
    E. Low dose of the prescribed drug

37. **Which of the following is NOT a feature of alcoholic hallucinosis?**
    A. Clear consciousness
    B. Autonomic hyperactivity
    C. Third-person hallucinations
    D. Secondary delusions
    E. Good prognosis compared with other psychoses

38. **An 18-year-old boy was brought to the A&E by police after being picked up wandering near Tower Bridge. He was angry, agitated, and suspicious. He was concerned about people trying to 'get him'. On examination, he showed evidence of stereotyped behaviour, tachycardia, pupillary dilation and elevated blood pressure. Soon after initial evaluation, he developed seizures. What is the most likely substance that may have led to this presentation?**
    A. Alcohol
    B. Cannabis
    C. Heroin
    D. Amphetamine
    E. Inhalant

39. **Cocaine intake is associated with all of the following phenomena except**
    A. Dopamine reuptake inhibition
    B. Serotonin reuptake inhibition
    C. Noradrenaline reuptake inhibition
    D. Corticotrophin releasing hormone secretion
    E. Prolactin release

40. **Martin has been admitted to the addictions unit to undergo detoxification from opiates. He has been known to suffer from low blood pressure. Which of the following would be the best agent to treat his withdrawal symptoms?**
    A. Buprenorphine
    B. Naloxone
    C. Clonidine
    D. Dihydrocodeine
    E. Lofexidine

41. **Tolerance doesn't develop to which of the following symptoms/signs in opiate dependence?**
    A. Sedation
    B. Euphoria
    C. Constipation
    D. Miosis
    E. Insomnia

42. **Donna is an active opiate user, who recently found out that she is pregnant. She approaches her GP saying she wants to stop her substance use and is not considering maintenance therapy with methadone. She is worried about withdrawal symptoms. Her GP calls you about the best time for Donna to undergo opiate withdrawal during pregnancy. Which of the following is the most appropriate answer?**
    A. First trimester
    B. Second trimester
    C. Third trimester
    D. Any of the above
    E. Withdrawal should never be considered during pregnancy

43. **Which of the following symptoms is NOT found in opiate withdrawal?**
    A. Abdominal pain
    B. Dry eyes
    C. Dilated pupils
    D. Vomiting
    E. Sweating

44. **Which of the following treatments for opioid dependence has been shown to reduce risk-taking behaviours associated with HIV transmission?**
    A. Naltrexone use
    B. Methadone maintenance
    C. Narcotics anonymous programme
    D. Antidepressant treatment
    E. Oral morphine prescription

45. **The half life of methadone in a patient with opioid dependence is**
    A. 4–6 hours
    B. 10–20 hours
    C. 24–36 hours
    D. 72–90 hours
    E. None of the above

46. **Which of the receptors is implicated in the respiratory depressant action of opioids?**

    A. Mu
    B. Kappa
    C. Delta
    D. Sigma
    E. ORL1

47. **What is the equivalent dose of methadone for 0.5 g of street heroin?**

    A. 5–15 mL of 1 mg/mL mixture
    B. 10–20 mL of 1 mg/mL mixture
    C. 30–40 mL of 1 mg/mL mixture
    D. 80–100 mL of 1 mg/ml mixture
    E. 1–2 mL of 1mg/mL mixture

48. **Amotivational syndrome has been described with the use of which of the following substance?**

    A. Cocaine
    B. Amphetamine
    C. Cannabis
    D. Alcohol
    E. LSD

49. **Maternal smoking during pregnancy has been best associated with which of the following?**

    A. Learning disability
    B. Autistic spectrum disorder
    C. Conduct disorder
    D. Autism
    E. Mood disorders

50. **Following recent consumption of LSD, it can be detected in urine for up to**

    A. 24 hours
    B. 1–3 days
    C. 10–15 days
    D. 15–30 days
    E. More than 30 days

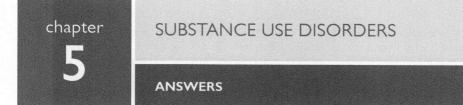
1. C.   According to Jellinek, drinking behaviour is heterogeneous. He described five species of alcoholism. Type *alpha* represents a purely habitual use without loss of control. A person with alpha alcoholism retains the ability to abstain. Type *beta* refers to development of physical complications without physical or psychological dependence. Type *gamma* represents acquired tissue tolerance leading to physical dependence and loss of control. They still maintain the ability to abstain if necessary. Type *delta* shares the three features of gamma, but the inability to abstain becomes prominent. Type *epsilon* refers to dipsomania or periodic alcoholism. More recently, various investigators have come up with different classifications, which overlap each other.

Murray R, *et al*, eds. *Essential Psychiatry*, 4th edn. Cambridge University Press, 2008, p. 198.
Sadock BJ and Sadock VA. *Kaplan and Sadock's Synopsis of Psychiatry: Behavioral Sciences/Clinical Psychiatry*, 10th edn. Lippincott Williams and Wilkins, 2007, p. 397.

2. E.   In 1976, Edwards and Gross proposed that not all people who drink too much are dependent on alcohol. They suggested the criteria for an alcohol dependence syndrome. This model forms the basis for the current ICD-10 classification. They noted that dependence was not an 'all or none' phenomenon, but lay on a spectrum of severity. The criteria were based on the clinical observation that some of the heavy drinkers manifested an interrelated clustering of signs and symptoms. The criteria are narrowing of repertoire; salience of drinking; increased tolerance to alcohol; withdrawal symptoms; relief drinking; subjective awareness of compulsion to drink; reinstatement after abstinence. Not all the elements need always be present, nor always present with the same intensity.

Murray RM, *et al*. *Essential Psychiatry*, 4th edn. Cambridge University Press; 2008, p. 198.

3. A.   ICD-10 includes six items under dependence, most of which are similar to DSM-IV. For a diagnosis of dependence, three or more items should have occurred in the past year. The 'strong desire or sense of compulsion to take the substance' is viewed as a central descriptive characteristic of dependence in ICD-10. This compulsive-use indicator is not included in the concept of dependence described by DSM-IV. DSM-IV also allows categorization of substance dependence with or without physiological dependence depending on the presence of tolerance and withdrawal symptoms.

Gelder MG, *et al*., eds. *New Oxford Textbook of Psychiatry*. Oxford University Press, 2000, p. 485.

4. A.   Alcohol dependence occurs in 15–20% of hospitalized patients in some settings. Hence withdrawal from alcohol is also a common presentation in this population. Withdrawal symptoms are minor in most cases, but they can be considerable and even fatal in some. Alcohol withdrawal delirium, commonly known as delirium tremens or 'DTs', is the most serious manifestation of alcohol withdrawal syndrome. Classic studies quote a mortality of around 15%, but with advances in treatment, mortality rates have fallen, and more recent studies indicate a mortality of 0 to 1% in treated cases.

Mayo-Smith MF, Beecher LH, Fischer TL, *et al*. Management of alcohol withdrawal delirium: an evidence-based practice guideline. *Archives of Internal Medicine* 2004; **164**: 1405–1412.

5. C.   Clinical features of alcohol withdrawal syndrome can appear within hours of the last drink (usually 6–12 hours) but alcohol withdrawal delirium typically does not develop until 2–3 days after cessation of drinking. Delirium tremens usually lasts 48–72 hours, but can last longer in some cases. Current diagnostic criteria for withdrawal delirium include disturbance of consciousness, change in cognition or perceptual disturbance developing in a short period, and the emergence of symptoms during or shortly after withdrawal from heavy alcohol intake. The classic clinical presentation also includes hyperpyrexia, tachycardia, hypertension, and diaphoresis. The neurobiological basis for withdrawal is a gradual upregulation of *N*-methyl-D-aspartate receptors under the influence of chronic alcohol use.

Mayo-Smith MF, Beecher LH, Fischer TL, *et al*. Management of alcohol withdrawal delirium: an evidence-based practice guideline. *Archives of Internal Medicine* 2004; **164**: 1405–1412.

6. E.   This question looks at the possible differential diagnoses in a case of alcohol-related seizure. All the given choices are results of laboratory investigations that may give us a clue of the possible cause for the seizure. Electrolyte imbalance, hypoglycaemia, subdural haematoma, and other substances in blood may be associated with an alcohol-induced seizure. EEG is useful in the setting of the first alcohol withdrawal seizure or where epilepsy is suspected, but not immediately after a seizure when a record of slow delta activity is found whatever the cause of the seizure. However, the inter-ictal EEG is usually within normal limits in alcohol withdrawal seizures, whereas a generalized spike and wave (epileptiform activity) patterns on the EEG points towards generalized epilepsy. Alcohol-related seizures do not predispose to epilepsy.

McKeon A, Frye MA and Delanty N. The alcohol withdrawal syndrome. *Journal of Neurology, Neurosurgery, and Psychiatry* 2008; **79**: 854–862.

7. C.   Benzodiazepines are the first-line treatment in alcohol withdrawal seizures. Lorazepam has been found to be superior to placebo in double-blind placebo-controlled studies of patients with chronic alcohol abuse presenting with a generalized seizure. The European treatment guidelines recommend either diazepam or lorazepam, although lorazepam is recommended over diazepam in the setting of status epilepticus. This is because lorazepam (although it has a shorter half-life than diazepam) maintains a steady plasma state for a longer time than diazepam, which is lipid soluble. The plasma levels of diazepam drop rapidly due to redistribution to fat. Placebo-controlled trials have demonstrated phenytoin to be ineffective in the secondary prevention of alcohol withdrawal seizures.

McKeon A, Frye MA and Delanty N. The alcohol withdrawal syndrome. *Journal of Neurology, Neurosurgery, and Psychiatry* 2008; **79**: 854–862.

8. D. General guidelines on the management of alcohol withdrawal advise against the use of neuroleptic agents as the sole pharmacological agents in the setting of delirium tremens, as they are associated with a longer duration of delirium, higher complication rate, and, ultimately, a higher mortality. However, neuroleptic agents have a role as a selected adjunct to benzodiazepines when agitation, thought disorder, or perceptual disturbances are not sufficiently controlled by benzodiazepines. Although haloperidol is well established in this setting, chlorpromazine is contraindicated as it is more epileptogenic. There is little information available on atypical antipsychotics in this regard.

Mayo-Smith MF, Beecher LH, Fischer TL, *et al.* Management of alcohol withdrawal delirium. An evidence-based practice guideline. *Archives of Internal Medicine* 2004; **164**: 1405–1412. McKeon A, Frye MA and Delanty N. The alcohol withdrawal syndrome. *Journal of Neurology, Neurosurgery, and Psychiatry* 2008; **79**: 854–862.

9. C. Failure to identify or consider Wernicke's encephalopathy, and failure to institute adequate thiamine replacement therapy, has an associated mortality of 20%. Wernicke's encephalopathy is an acute neuropsychiatric condition associated with biochemical brain lesion caused by the depletion of intracellular thiamine (vitamin B1). Although reversible in the early stages, continued depletion leads to cellular energy deficit, focal acidosis, regional increase in glutamate, and ultimately cell death. Ninety per cent of the cases in developed countries are associated with alcohol misuse. This deficiency may be due to dietary deficiency, reduced absorption, and the increased excretion of thiamine seen in alcohol users. Clinical features include delirium with prominent anterograde amnesia, ataxia, and ophthalmoplegia. Imaging may reveal the presence of small haemorrhages in mamillary bodies and thalami.

Thomson AD and Marshall EJ. The natural history and pathophysiology of Wernicke's encephalopathy and Korsakoff's psychosis. *Alcohol Alcohol* 2006; **41**: 151–158.

10. E. Seventy-five per cent of cases with Wernicke's encephalopathy will be left with permanent brain damage involving severe short-term memory loss (Korsakoff's dementia) if adequate parenteral therapy with thiamine is not instituted. In clinical practice, Wernicke's encephalopathy may be difficult to recognize because all the classic symptoms may not be present. In addition, the symptoms may be coloured by the presence of other comorbidities such as withdrawal delirium or seizures. Some authors also suggest the presence of a subsyndromal version of the encephalopathy that may present only with minor symptoms and neuroimaging findings. Twenty-five per cent of patients with Korsakoff's dementia will require long-term institutionalization.

Thomson AD and Marshall EJ. The natural history and pathophysiology of Wernicke's Encephalopathy and Korsakoff's Psychosis. *Alcohol Alcohol* 2006; **41**: 151–8.

11. C. Risk factors for developing Wernicke's encephalopathy include a greater degree of malnutrition and severity of alcohol misuse. Oral thiamine hydrochloride cannot be relied on to provide adequate thiamine to patients at risk. This is because studies show that only a maximum of 4.5 mg of thiamine will be absorbed from an oral dose over 30 mg. In addition, patients with alcohol problems tend to have poor absorption. Therefore, intravenous delivery of high-potency B-complex vitamin therapy containing thiamine remains the standard of care for those patients with suspected Wernicke's encephalopathy (500 mg of thiamine three times daily for three days), or who are at risk for Wernicke's encephalopathy (250 mg three times daily for 3–5 days). In the outpatient setting, the administration of a course of intramuscular thiamine 200 mg for 5 days has been recommended because the absorption of thiamine is negated further by continued drinking after hospital discharge.

Thomson AD, Cook CC, Touquet R, et al. The Royal College of Physicians report on alcohol: guidelines for managing Wernicke's encephalopathy in the Accident and Emergency Department. Alcohol Alcohol 2002; **37**: 513–521.

12. B. Up to 40% of people with an alcohol use disorder attempt suicide at some time and 7% end their lives by committing suicide. Risk factors include being male, older than 50 years of age, living alone, being unemployed, poor social support, interpersonal losses, continued drinking, consumption of a greater amount of alcohol when drinking, a recent alcohol binge, previous alcohol treatment, a family history of alcoholism, a history of comorbid substance abuse (especially cocaine), a major depressive episode, serious medical illness, and prior suicidal behaviour. Suicidal behaviour is especially frequent in patients with comorbid alcoholism and major depression.

Sher L. Risk and protective factors for suicide in patients with alcoholism. Scientific World Journal 2006; **6**: 1405–1411.

13. A. Alcohol use disorder co-occurs with other major mental illnesses. The Epidemiology Catchment Area Study reported a 13.8% lifetime prevalence for alcohol abuse or dependence in persons with bipolar I disorder in the US general population. Lifetime prevalence of alcohol abuse or dependence are: bipolar I, 46.2%; bipolar II, 39.2%; schizophrenia, 33.7%; panic disorder, 28.7%; unipolar depression, 16.5%. Patients with mania had an odds ratio of 6.2 (highest) for co-occurring alcohol abuse and/or dependence. Considering the degree of psychiatric comorbidity among alcohol-dependent individuals, the National Comorbidity Survey showed that the odds ratio (OR) of having co-occurring lifetime diagnosis of mania in patients with a lifetime diagnosis of alcohol dependence was higher in both men (OR = 12.03) and women (OR = 5.3).

Regier DA, Farmer ME, Rae DS, et al. Comorbidity of mental disorders with alcohol and other drug abuse. Results from the Epidemiologic Catchment Area (ECA) Study. Journal of the American Medical Association 1990; **264**: 2511–2518.

Kessler RC, Crum RM, Warner LA, et al. Lifetime co-occurrence of DSM-III-R alcohol abuse and dependence with other psychiatric disorders in the National Comorbidity Survey. Archives of General Psychiatry 1997; **54**: 313–321.

Fan AH FM, Masseling SJ, et al. Increased suicidality in mania complicated by alcoholism. Psychiatry and Clinical Neuroscience 2007; **4**: 34–39.

14. C. This question can be answered using results from a study called Project MATCH (Matching Alcoholism Treatments to Client Heterogeneity). MATCH is one of the largest randomized trials to have examined psychosocial interventions for people with alcohol-related problems. The study is a multicentric study that involved randomizing over 1700 patients to MET, CBT, or TSF. This study demonstrated that four sessions of MET were as effective for treating alcohol dependence as 12 sessions of CBT or TSF therapy. The benefits from treatment persisted for up to 3 years. Clients with a higher degree of baseline anger fared better with MET than CBT or TSF. MET was found to be more cost-effective than CBT or TSF.

The Project MATCH study and smaller patient-matching studies provide support for the effectiveness of TSF programmes. Patients in Project MATCH who received outpatient TSF were most likely to abstain from alcohol during the first post-treatment year. TSF therapy led to a greater length of time before the patient's first relapse and to a higher percentage of abstinent patients at 1- and 3-year follow-up. Patients in Project MATCH with social networks supportive of not drinking responded better to TSF than MET, and that participation in AA was a mediator of this effect. Project MATCH found that patients who were rated high in 'meaning-seeking' fared better with TSF than CBT and MET at 1-year follow-up.

Tyrer P and Silk KR. *Cambridge Textbook of Effective Treatments in Psychiatry*, 1st edn. Cambridge University Press; 2008, p. 274.

15. A. Brief interventions are recommended for reduction of alcohol use for patients across age and gender who are heavy or problem drinkers and do not meet the criteria for severe alcohol dependence. Brief interventions are intended to be conducted by health professionals who usually are not involved in addiction treatment, e.g. clinicians in general medical and other primary care settings. Brief interventions may differ in intensity from a single 5-minute session of simple advice to stop drinking to multiple sessions lasting up to 60 minutes each. They generally consist of four or fewer visits. They are generally useful for the prevention of alcohol-related problems in patients who are at risk of developing them. They are not primarily used as a maintenance therapy for fully fledged alcohol use disorders like dependence. The content of brief interventions can be remembered using the acronym FRAMES developed by Miller and Rollnick: *feedback* about the adverse effects of alcohol; emphasis on personal *responsibility* for changing the dysfunctional behaviour; *advice* about reducing or abstaining from the behaviour; a *menu* of options for further help; *empathic stance* towards the patient; and an emphasis on *self-efficacy*.

Gelder MG *et al.*, eds. *New Oxford Textbook of Psychiatry*. Oxford University Press, 2000, p. 270.

16. C. In the United Kingdom, a unit is 8 grams of pure alcohol, equivalent to half a pint of ordinary beer, a small glass of wine (9% strength), or one measure of spirits. In the USA a single drink is usually considered to contain about 12 grams of ethanol, which is the content of 12 ounces of beer, one 4-ounce glass of non-fortified wine, or 1–1.5 ounces of 40% ethanol liquor (e.g. whiskey or gin). Using moderate sizes of drinks, clinicians estimate that a single 'drink' (1.5 units) increases the blood alcohol level of a 150-pound man by 15–20 mg/dL, which is about the concentration of alcohol that an average person can metabolize in 1 hour.

Murray RM, Kendler KS, McGuffin P, *et al. Essential Psychiatry*, 4th edn. Cambridge University Press, 2008, p. 199.

17. C. Nearly 90% of alcohol is absorbed from small intestine, with the remaining 10% absorbed from the stomach. Alcohol reaches peak blood concentration approximately 45–60 minutes after consumption. Absorption is enhanced by an empty stomach whereas food delays absorption. When the alcohol concentration in the stomach becomes too high, gastric mucus secretion increases, leading to closure of the pyloric valve. This pylorospasm slows down the absorption and protects from rapid intoxication but can lead to vomiting and nausea in drinkers.

The intoxicating effects are greater when the blood alcohol concentration is rising than when it is falling; this is called the Mellanby effect. As a result, the rate of absorption directly affects the intoxication response. Nearly 90% of absorbed alcohol is metabolized through oxidation in the liver; the remainder is excreted unchanged by the kidneys and lungs. The rate of oxidation by the liver is constant (15 mg/dL per hour) and independent of plasma alcohol levels; thus alcohol follows zero-order elimination kinetics. Women have a tendency to become more intoxicated than men after drinking the same amount of alcohol; this may be due to differences in absorption kinetics and a lower level of metabolic enzymes such as alcohol dehydrogenase (ADH) in women.

Sadock BJ and Sadock VA. *Kaplan and Sadock's Synopsis of Psychiatry: Behavioral Sciences/Clinical Psychiatry*, 10th edn. Lippincott Williams and Wilkins, 2007, p. 393.

18. A. AUDIT is a 10-item questionnaire, covering quantity, frequency, inability to control drinking, withdrawal relief, loss of memory, injury, and concern by others. A score of 8 or more indicates that the person is drinking to a degree that is harmful or hazardous, whereas a score of 13 or more in women and 15 or more in men is indicative of dependent drinking. It is a very useful and widely used scale. The CAGE questionnaire is a simple, easily administered instrument that has only four items. A positive answer should raise suspicion of an alcohol problem, and a score of 2 is highly suggestive of one. It takes 30–120 seconds to administer. Aertgeerts *et al* studied alcohol screening instruments used in general practice. They found that CAGE was an insufficient screening instrument for detecting alcohol misuse or dependence among primary care patients with only 62% sensitivity for males and 54% for females. AUDIT was found to be more effective, with a sensitivity of 83% among males and 65% among females. However, this was using a cut off-point of 5 rather than the usual 8. The study also found that conventional laboratory tests are of no use for detecting alcohol abuse or dependence in a primary care setting. MAST is the Michigan alcohol screening test and the other options in the question are laboratory-based blood tests.

Aertgeerts B, Buntix F, Ansoms S and Fevery J. (2001) Screening properties of questionnaires and laboratory tests for the detection of alcohol abuse or dependence in a general practice population. *British Journal of General Practice* **51**: 206–217.

19. A. Alcohol-related blackouts are similar to episodes of transient global amnesia; they occur as discrete episodes of anterograde amnesia in association with alcohol intoxication. Despite a specific short-term memory deficit (inability to recall events that happened in the previous 5–10 minutes) during the blackouts and significant subjective distress that follows, patients have relatively intact remote memory and can perform complicated tasks during a blackout. Thus they appear completely normal to casual observers. It is thought that alcohol blocks the consolidation of new memories into old memories via its action on medial temporal structures. Binge drinkers may be particularly prone to alcoholic blackouts due to repeated intoxications. Although amnesia may accompany withdrawal or intoxication-related generalized seizures, not all blackouts are associated with epileptic activity in EEG.

Sadock BJ and Sadock VA. *Kaplan and Sadock's Synopsis of Psychiatry: Behavioral Sciences/Clinical Psychiatry*, 10th edn. Lippincott Williams and Wilkins, 2007, p. 400.

20. A.   Children with FAS commonly present with microcephaly rather than macrocephaly. It is well documented that alcohol and its metabolite acetaldehyde can have serious effects on the developing foetus. Currently, the estimated incidence of FAS is between 1 and 3 cases per 1000 live births. It is one of the most frequent causes of birth defects associated with learning disability, and the most common of non-hereditary causes of birth defects. Clinical features of FAS include prenatal and postnatal growth retardation, central nervous system abnormalities, usually with learning disability (up to severe), a characteristic facial dysmorphism (e.g., absent philtrum, flattened nasal bridge, short palpebral fissures, epicanthic folds, and maxillary hypoplasia), and an array of other birth defects such as microcephaly, altered palmar creases, short stature, syndactyly, atrial septal defect and other heart abnormalities. Full-blown foetal alcohol syndrome is seen in the offspring of approximately one-third of alcoholic women drinking the equivalent of 10–15 units daily. It is also more common in women who binge drink.

Lowinson JH, Ruiz P, Millman RB and Langrod JG. *Substance Abuse: A Comprehensive Textbook*, 4th edn. Lippincott Williams & Wilkins, 2005, p. 1052.

21. C.   Sedative-hypnotic (includes benzodiazepines, barbiturates and newer 'z' hypnotics) withdrawal syndrome is a spectrum of signs and symptoms that occurs after stopping daily intake of a sedative-hypnotic. Common signs and symptoms include anxiety, tremors, nightmares, insomnia, anorexia, nausea, vomiting, postural hypotension, seizures, delirium, and hyperpyrexia. The withdrawal syndrome is similar for all sedative-hypnotics, but the severity and time course depend on the pharmacokinetics of the individual agent used, besides a number of other risk factors. With short-acting medication, withdrawal symptoms typically begin 12–24 hours after the last dose and peak in intensity between 24 and 72 hours after the last dose. If the patient has liver disease or is over the age of 65, symptoms may develop more slowly. With long-acting medication, the withdrawal syndrome usually begins 24 to 48 hours after the last dose and peaks on the fifth to eighth day. During untreated sedative-hypnotic withdrawal, the EEG may show bursts of *high-voltage, low-frequency activity*. This may precede a clinical seizure occasionally.

Lowinson JH, Ruiz P, Millman RB and Langrod JG. *Substance Abuse: A Comprehensive Textbook*. 4th edn. Lippincott Williams & Wilkins, 2005, p. 307.

22. A.   ADH (alcohol dehydrogenase) and ALDH (aldehyde dehydrogenase) are the major enzymes involved in the degradation of ethanol; ADH catabolizes alcohol to acetaldehyde, which ALDH breaks down to acetate and water. A number of studies have shown that allelic variants of ADH and ALDH are associated with the risk for developing alcohol dependence. There are many ALDH gene families distributed on several different chromosomes. Family 2 genes (ALDH 2) located on chromosome 12 have been studied the most regarding an association with alcohol dependence. This family of genes encodes mitochondrial enzymes that oxidize acetaldehyde. ALDH 2 has an allelic variant called ALDH 2*2. This ALDH 2*2 variant is found in approximately 50% of the Asian population. Individuals with the ALDH 2*2 variant typically experience a disulfiram-like reaction when they take alcohol. This is sometimes called the 'Asian flush' or the 'Oriental flush syndrome'. Several studies demonstrate the protective effect of ALDH 2*2 gene carriers from developing alcohol dependence. The other genes ALDH1, 3, 4 and 5 are responsible for the metabolism of other aldehydes in the body. Similarly a variant allele of the ADH gene (situated on chromosome 4) ADH 2*2 also confers protection to alcoholism, although this relationship is less robust than ALDH2*2.

Lowinson JH, Ruiz P, Millman RB and Langrod JG. *Substance Abuse: A Comprehensive Textbook*, 4th edn. Lippincott Williams & Wilkins, 2005, p. 37.

23. C. About 30–40% of people with an alcohol-related disorder meet the diagnostic criteria for a major depressive disorder sometime during their lifetime. It is more common in women. It is dose dependent, i.e. it is likely to occur in patients who have a high daily consumption of alcohol. It is also more common in those with a family history of alcohol abuse. Patients with depression and comorbid alcohol use disorders are at a greater risk for attempting/completing suicide and are likely to have other substance-related disorder diagnoses. Most estimates of the prevalence of suicide among people with alcohol-related disorders range from 10–15%, although alcohol use itself may be involved in a much higher percentage of suicides. Twenty to 50 percent of all people with alcohol-related disorders also meet the diagnostic criteria for an anxiety disorder. Phobias and panic disorder are particularly frequent comorbid diagnoses in patients with alcohol use disorders.

Sadock BJ and Sadock VA. *Kaplan and Sadock's Synopsis of Psychiatry: Behavioral Sciences/Clinical Psychiatry*, 10th edn. Lippincott Williams and Wilkins, 2007, p. 392.

24. E. Acamprosate's principal neurochemical effects have been attributed to antagonism of NMDA glutamate receptors, which restores the balance between excitatory and inhibitory neurotransmission that is dysregulated following chronic alcohol consumption. Recently, however, further mechanisms have been demonstrated. Thus acamprosate is said to have four principal effects: A) reducing post-synaptic excitatory amino acid neurotransmission at N-methyl-D-aspartate (NMDA); B) diminishing Ca^{2+} influx into the cell, which interferes with expression of the immediate early gene c-fos; C) decreasing the sensitivity of voltage-gated calcium channels, and D) modulating metabotropic-5 glutamate receptors (mGluR5). The most common side effects are headache, diarrhoea, flatulence, abdominal pain, paraesthesias, and various skin reactions. Acamprosate is not metabolised by liver and is excreted unchanged by the kidney. Administration of disulfiram or diazepam does not affect the pharmacokinetics of acamprosate. Coadministration of naltrexone with acamprosate produces an increase in concentrations of acamprosate. Effect of acamprosate is dose dependent and has been confirmed by at least two studies in humans.

Johnson BA. Update on neuropharmacological treatments for alcoholism: scientific basis and clinical findings. *Biochemical Pharmacology* 2008; **75**: 34–56.

Pelc I, Verbanck P, Le Bon O, *et al.* Efficacy and safety of acamprosate in the treatment of detoxified alcohol-dependent patients. A 90-day placebo-controlled dose-finding study. *British Journal of Psychiatry* 1997; **171**: 73–77.

25. D. Disulfiram inhibits aldehyde dehydrogenase producing a marked increase in blood acetaldehyde concentration if alcohol is consumed. The accumulation of acetaldehyde produces a wide array of unpleasant reactions, called the disulfiram–ethanol reaction, characterized by nausea, throbbing headache, vomiting, hypertension, flushing, sweating, thirst, dyspnoea, tachycardia, chest pain, vertigo, and blurred vision. The reaction occurs almost immediately after the ingestion of one alcoholic drink and can last from 30 minutes to 2 hours. A person taking disulfiram must be instructed that the ingestion/use of any quantity of alcohol (including alcohol-containing preparations of medicines, food, and cosmetics) would lead to the unpleasant reaction with dangerous consequences at times. Disulfiram should not be administered until the person has abstained from alcohol for at least 12 hours. This reaction can occur as long as 1–2 weeks after the last dose of disulfiram.

Sadock BJ and Sadock VA. *Kaplan and Sadock's Synopsis of Psychiatry: Behavioral Sciences/clinical Psychiatry*, 10th edn. Lippincott Williams & Wilkins, 2007, p. 1038.

26. C. Learned tolerance refers to a reduction in the effects of a drug because of compensatory mechanisms that are acquired by past experiences. One type of learned tolerance is called *behavioural tolerance*. This simply describes the skills that can be developed through repeated experiences of attempting to function despite a state of mild to moderate intoxication. A common example is learning to walk in a straight line despite the motor impairment produced by alcohol intoxication. This probably involves both acquisition of motor skills and the learned awareness of one's deficit, causing the person to walk more carefully. At higher levels of intoxication, behavioural tolerance is overcome, and the deficits are obvious. Pharmacokinetic, or dispositional, tolerance refers to changes in the distribution or metabolism of a drug after repeated administrations such that a given dose produces a lower blood concentration than the same dose did on initial exposure. This may be mediated via enzyme induction. *Pharmacodynamic tolerance* refers to adaptive changes that have taken place within the systems affected by the drug so that the response to a given concentration of the drug is reduced, e.g. change in receptor density. *Conditioned tolerance* is the process where environmental cues, e.g. sight, smell, etc, for the substance will no longer produce a manifestation of the drug's effect. *Reverse tolerance,* or *sensitization,* refers to an increase in response with repetition of the same dose of the drug.

Zack M and Vogel-Sprott M. Behavioral tolerance and sensitization to alcohol in humans: the contribution of learning. *Experimental and Clinical Psychopharmacology* 1995; **3**: 396–401.

27. D. Miller and Rollnick (1991) described five principles that are essential to motivational interviewing. They are (1) express empathy: communicate acceptance, use reflective listening, and normalize a client's ambivalence; (2) develop discrepancy: increase the client's awareness of the consequences of the problematic behaviour, orient the client to the discrepancy between his/her current behaviour and goals in life, and have the client generate reasons for change; (3) avoid argumentation; (4) roll with resistance: invite the client to consider new points of view rather than having them imposed; and (5) support self-efficacy.

O'Donohue WT, Fisher JE and Hayes SC. Cognitive Behavior Therapy: *Applying Empirically Supported Techniques in Your Practice*. John Wiley & Sons; 2003, p. 252.

28. B. Although the occurrence of alcoholic hallucinosis has been noted for centuries, its nosological status is not yet clear. Little research regarding this has been published in recent years. Tsuang *et al.* (1994) reported a prevalence of 7.4% among patients in an alcohol treatment programme. Patients with alcoholic hallucinosis were younger at the onset of alcohol problems, consumed more alcohol per occasion, developed more alcohol-related life problems, had higher rates of drug experimentation, and used more of other drugs than alcohol users without hallucinosis. The severity of dependence increased the risk for hallucinosis. It is also noted that the prevalence of schizophrenia is higher in the families of index cases with alcoholic hallucinosis.

Tsuang JW, Irwin MR, Smith TL and Schuckit MA. Characteristics of men with alcoholic hallucinosis. *Addiction* 1994; **89**: 73–78.
Thirthalli J and Benegal V. Psychosis among substance users. *Current Opinions in Psychiatry* **19**: 239–245.

29. B. Decreased D2 receptors in alcohol, cocaine, and methamphetamine users, whether premorbid or the consequence of substance use, in conjunction with a finding of increased salience to drug cues, indicate susceptibility to relapse in this population.

Chang L and Haning W. Insights from recent positron emission tomographic studies of drug abuse and dependence. *Current Opinions in Psychiatry* **19**: 246–252.

30. B. Genetic and familial factors probably account for most cases of alcohol problems that begin in adulthood and continue through to older age. Late-onset cases are associated with much lower rates of family alcoholism. Compared with early-onset cases, late-onset problem drinkers also tend to have less psychopathology. In fact, the notion that late-onset alcohol dependence usually occurs secondary to a mood or organic mental disorder has not been upheld in recent systematic studies. The inability to cope with major losses, chronic psychosocial strains, or transient negative affects such as depression or loneliness, are associated with new or renewed problem drinking. The pathophysiological effects of alcohol may be more serious in elderly people because of an age-related increase in biological sensitivity to alcohol and in peak blood level following a standard alcohol load. In addition, alcohol also aggravates many pre-existing diseases that are more common in later life.

Gelder MG, et al., eds. *New Oxford Textbook of Psychiatry*. Oxford University Press, 2000, p. 1638.

31. C. The stages of change model by Prochaska and DiClemente are stages that a person goes through when involved in a behavioural change. This may include a change in substance misuse behaviour, starting daily exercise, going on a diet, or changing a health-related behaviour, e.g. attempting to obtain a cervical smear. The first stage is the precontemplation stage, where the person is not thinking of any imminent change and is happy the way things are. The second stage is contemplation, where he is considering a change in the near future. Preparation is when he gets ready or prepares to enforce the behavioural change. The action phase is when he implements the change, and in the maintenance phase he decides to continue the change in behaviour and attempts to prevent relapse.

Thambirajah MS. *Psychological Basis of Psychiatry*. Elsevier, 2005, pp. 125–126.

32. E. Disulfiram is generally considered a deterrent. Earlier works suggested disulfiram to be an aversion treatment. The theory underlying 'aversion therapy' is that 'repeated pairing' of alcohol with an unpleasant stimulus leads to a conditioned response in which drinking alcohol is increasingly perceived as unpleasant. This was previously considered to be the case with disulfiram, because it was common practice to induce the highly unpleasant but controlled disulfiram–ethanol reaction in a clinical setting before initiating regular therapy. This is now considered unnecessary for the efficacy of disulfiram therapy, i.e. the 'unpleasant' outcome need not be experienced by the person, but a 'fear' of the possibility of such experience is sufficient. An analogy is with police cars. Brewer states that no sane driver will exceed the speed limit if he sees a police car in front or behind; one does not need to be arrested for speeding before reducing the speed. Most patients who take disulfiram under supervision do not risk drinking. Those who do drink do not necessarily get a significant reaction on standard doses of disulfiram, but if the experience is unpleasant, they do not usually repeat it. Some people may consider this as a form of negative reinforcement, which again needs the subject to experience the 'repeated conditioning' in order to increase the abstinence behaviour. So, from the given choices, deterrence theory would be the best choice. Deterrence is an established theme in criminal justice. It refers to reduction in unwanted behaviour through knowledge of costs and risks involved in an act.

Brewer C. Combining pharmacological antagonists and behavioural psychotherapy in treating addictions. Why it is effective but unpopular? *British Journal of Psychiatry* 1990; **157**: 34–40.

33. A. High doses of cocaine have been associated with a wide variety of toxic effects, including cardiac arrhythmias, coronary artery spasms, myocardial infarction, and myocarditis. Most of the complications are related to vasoconstriction. The most common cerebrovascular diseases associated with cocaine use are non-haemorrhagic cerebral infarctions. When haemorrhagic infarctions do occur, they can include subarachnoid, intraparenchymal, intraventricular, and at times spinal cord haemorrhages. Other toxic effects on the central nervous system may include seizures, hyperpyrexia, respiratory depression, and death. Cocaine-related seizures and loss of consciousness are seen in heavy users. Rhabdomyolysis, after large doses of cocaine, may contribute to renal complications. Sniffing cocaine can cause ulcers of the mucosa in the nose and perforation of the nasal septum from persistent vasoconstriction. Inhaled cocaine freebase is believed to induce lung damage. By producing placental vasoconstriction, cocaine may contribute to foetal anoxia.

Sadock BJ and Sadock VA. *Kaplan and Sadock's Comprehensive Textbook of Psychiatry*, 8th edn. Lippincott Williams and Wilkins, 2005, p. 1229.

34. B. Alcohol use disorders run in families. A child with an alcoholic parent has a 4- to 10-fold increased risk of developing alcoholism themselves. This can be due to both genetic and environmental factors. Environmental influences include the availability of alcohol, parental attitudes, and peer pressure. Starting to drink before the age of 15 years is associated with a fourfold increased risk for lifetime alcoholism compared with starting at the age of 21 years. Severe childhood stressors, especially emotional, physical, and sexual abuse, are associated with up to seven times increased risk of alcoholism in adulthood. Childhood antisocial behaviour predicts regular alcohol use in early adolescence and the development of alcoholism later on.

Enoch M. Genetic and environmental influences on the development of alcoholism: resilience vs. risk. *Annals of the New York Academy of Sciences* 2006; **1094**: 193–201.

35. A. Cocaine use is associated with frequent co-occurrence of other psychiatric disorders. The presence of other psychiatric disorders sharply increases the odds of substance dependence, and substance-dependent people are more likely than the general population to meet the diagnostic criteria for additional psychiatric disorders. Among cocaine users seeking treatment, the rates of additional current and lifetime diagnoses are regularly found to be elevated. The most common additional lifetime diagnoses associated with cocaine use are alcoholism (60%), antisocial personality (30%), and major depression (30%).

Sadock BJ and Sadock VA. *Kaplan and Sadock's Comprehensive Textbook of Psychiatry*, 8th edn. Lippincott Williams and Wilkins, 2005, p. 1228.

36. D. Symptoms associated with the withdrawal of benzodiazepine therapy may reflect one of three phenomena – a recurrence (return of the original symptoms); a rebound (worsening of the original symptoms), or true withdrawal (emergence of new symptoms). These symptoms may include anxiety, dysphoria, irritability, altered sleep–wake cycle, daytime drowsiness, tachycardia, elevated blood pressure, hyperreflexia, muscle tension, agitation/motor restlessness, tremor, myoclonus, muscle and joint pain. Patients may also experience various perceptual disturbances such as hyperacusis, depersonalization, blurred vision, and hallucinations. In severe cases, delirium similar to delirium tremens has been reported. Factors influencing the development of the discontinuance or withdrawal syndrome include the dose of the drug, duration of the drug intake, rapid tapering of the dose and greater psychopathology before initiation and termination of medication, dependent personality traits, and lower education levels.

Sadock BJ and Sadock VA. *Kaplan and Sadock's Comprehensive Textbook of Psychiatry*, 8th edn. Lippincott Williams and Wilkins, 2005, p. 1311.

37. B. Alcoholic hallucinosis is a condition in which auditory hallucinations are present during clear consciousness in the absence of autonomic overactivity, usually in a person who has been drinking excessively for many years. Initially the hallucinations are simple in nature, but later on become complex voices that are derogatory. These voices are usually second person, but at times are third person. They may also be command hallucinations. Delusions, if present are secondary to the voice. In both ICD-10 and DSM-IV, the disorder is classified as a substance-induced psychotic disorder. The differential diagnosis includes withdrawal symptoms and delirium tremens. In both these conditions the auditory hallucinations are transient and disorganized, and in the latter, consciousness is impaired. Auditory hallucinations of alcoholic hallucinosis are persistent and organized, and occur during clear consciousness. The hallucinations usually respond rapidly to antipsychotic medication. The prognosis is good; usually the condition improves within days or a couple of weeks, provided that the person remains abstinent. Symptoms that last for 6 months generally continue for years. The other differential diagnosis one needs to rule out, especially in the presence of derogatory hallucinations, is major depression with psychotic symptoms.

Gelder MG, et al., eds. New Oxford Textbook of Psychiatry. Oxford University Press, 2000, p. 490.

38. D. The features described in the clinical scenario are that of amphetamine intoxication. The clinching points are the sympathetic activity due to release of catecholamines and the stereotyped behaviour, which are characteristic of amphetamine use. According to DSM-IV, the diagnostic criteria for intoxication with amphetamine includes behavioural or psychological changes such as euphoria or affective blunting; changes in sociability; hypervigilance; interpersonal sensitivity; anxiety, tension, or anger; stereotyped behaviours; and impaired judgment. Physical symptoms/signs include tachycardia or bradycardia, pupillary dilation, elevated or lowered blood pressure, perspiration or chills with nausea or vomiting. Psychomotor changes include agitation or retardation. Patients may complain of muscular weakness, chest pain; some may develop cardiac arrhythmias and seizures.

Gelder MG. et al., eds. New Oxford Textbook of Psychiatry. Oxford University Press, 2000, p. 531.

39. E. Cocaine inhibits the normal reuptake of monoamines from the synaptic cleft by binding to transporter proteins. Its reinforcing effects are primarily due to its actions at the dopamine transporter, producing high levels of dopamine in the synapse. Cocaine also inhibits reuptake of noradrenaline and serotonin. The increase in noradrenaline concentration is important for some of cocaine's toxic effects. The drug produces increases in adrenocorticotropic hormone (ACTH) and cortisol by stimulating release of hypothalamic corticotropin-releasing hormone (CRH). Acutely, cocaine also stimulates the release of luteinizing hormone and follicle-stimulating hormone (FSH) and suppresses the release of prolactin.

Goldman D, Oroszi G and Ducci F. The genetics of addictions: uncovering the genes. Focus 2005; **4**: 401–415.

40. A. Buprenorphine is preferable to α2 adrenergic agonists if there are concerns about bradycardia or hypotension. Buprenorphine results in lower severity of withdrawal symptoms than α2 adrenergic agonists. Buprenorphine can be used for short-term opioid withdrawal and has a better outcome than clonidine. Methadone and α2 adrenergic agonists (e.g. clonidine and lofexidine) also have a good evidence base for reducing withdrawal symptoms. If a short duration of treatment is desirable, α2 adrenergic agonists are preferable to methadone. Methadone treatment is more successful if carried out slowly or with a linear dose reduction. Methadone can be used during pregnancy, and there are emerging studies regarding the use of buprenorphine. α2 adrenergic agonists should not be prescribed in pregnancy.

Lingford-Hughes AR, Welch S, Nutt DJ. Evidence-based guidelines for the pharmacological management of substance misuse, addiction and comorbidity: recommendations from the British Association for Psychopharmacology. Journal of Psychopharmacology 2004; **18**: 293–335.

41. C. Recent research has shed new light on the mechanisms involved in the development of opioid tolerance and dependence. Stimulation of opioid receptors located on critical cells such as those located in the locus coeruleus produces a decrease in cell firing. This effect reflects cellular hyperpolarization that results from both the activation of potassium channels and the inhibition of slowly depolarizing sodium channels. These actions occur in conjunction with a decrease in intracellular cyclic adenosine monophosphate (cAMP) levels. Among the given choices, both constipation and miosis have been traditionally thought to be resistant to tolerance. Kollars and Larson reviewed the two studies conducted in the late 60s which are often quoted to show that miosis does not develop tolerance. They quote a number of other studies which have shown that miosis is susceptible to tolerance. There are comparatively few data refuting the lack of tolerance response for constipation. Clinical experience hints that constipation is a major problem that persists without development of tolerance, especially in elderly people who are prescribed opiates as analgesics. This can be very difficult to treat, at times requiring enemas and in severe cases requiring manual evacuation.

Kollars JP and Larson M. tolerance to miotic effects of opioids. *Anesthesiology.* 2005; **102**: 701.
Higgins S, Stitzer M, McCaul M, *et al.* Pupillary response to methadone challenge in heroin users. *Clinical Pharmacology and Therapeutics* 1985; **37**: 460–463.

42. B. The view of treatment of opiate dependence has changed over the past 25 years. Previously it was thought that all patients should undergo withdrawal prior to delivery. Current practice acknowledges the fact that an abstinence state is almost impossible to achieve in this population. Hence most experts now advocate methadone maintenance as a way to reduce illegal drug use and remove the woman from a hazardous drug-seeking environment. Current consensus is that undertaking a medical withdrawal regimen could be accomplished most safely during the second trimester, with careful monitoring of foetal welfare by perinatal experts. The consensus is that opiate withdrawal could be best accomplished through stabilization with methadone followed by gradual reduction of the methadone dosage by 2–2.5 mg every 7–10 days. This should ideally be done only in a secondary care setting with the involvement of obstetricians and neonatologists.

Lowinson JH, Ruiz P, Millman RB and Langrod JG. *Substance Abuse: A Comprehensive Textbook*, 4th edn. Lippincott Williams & Wilkins, 2005, p. 808.

43. B. Lacrimation – not dry eyes – is a symptom seen in opiate withdrawal. DSM-IV states that opiate withdrawal can be precipitated by cessation of (or reduction in) opioid use that has been heavy and prolonged (several weeks or longer) or administration of an opioid antagonist after a period of opioid use. Other symptoms typically associated with withdrawal are dysphoric mood, nausea or vomiting, muscle aches, rhinorrhoea, pupillary dilation, piloerection, sweating, diarrhoea, yawning, fever, and insomnia. Piloerection along with general 'secretion' from most of the glands is called the 'cold turkey', when people tend to detox without medical help.

Sadock BJ and Sadock VA. *Kaplan and Sadock's Synopsis of Psychiatry: Behavioral Sciences/clinical Psychiatry*, 10th edn. Lippincott Williams & Wilkins, 2007, p. 447.

44. B. Systematic reviews of methadone maintenance vs. non-opioid therapy conducted by the Cochrane collaboration shows that methadone has a superior retention rate than control conditions. Methadone maintenance treatment has also been shown to reduce risk behaviours (specifically reduction in needle sharing) and thereby has achieved a reduction in the transmission of HIV. Intake of illicit opioids decreased in the methadone maintenance group, as shown by fewer positive urine tests for 'morphine' in these groups. Although criminal activity was found to be less in the group that was on methadone maintenance, the statistics did not show a significant difference. Nevertheless, individual randomized controlled trials have shown that methadone maintenance decreases criminal activity. In addition, methadone maintenance has shown to decrease rates of suicide and overdose in this population.

Mattick RP, Breen C, Kimber J, *et al.* Methadone maintenance therapy versus no opioid replacement therapy for opioid dependence. Cochrane Database of Systematic Reviews 2003, Issue 2. Art. No.: CD002209.

45. C. Elimination of most synthetic opioids is complex. The peak plasma concentrations of oral methadone are reached within 2–6 hours, and initially plasma half-life is 4–6 hours in opioid-naive people and 24–36 hours after steady dosing of any type of opioid. It generally requires once-daily dosing. Methadone is highly protein bound and equilibrates widely throughout the body, which ensures little post-dosage variation in steady-state plasma concentrations. Methadone can be used for short-term detoxification (7–30 days), long-term detoxification (up to 180 days), and maintenance (treatment beyond 180 days) of opioid-dependent individuals. In contrast, the elimination of a sublingual dosage of buprenorphine occurs in two phases: an initial phase with a half-life of 3–5 hours and a terminal phase with a half-life of more than 24 hours. Buprenorphine dissociates from its receptor binding site slowly, which permits an every-other-day dosing schedule.

Sadock BJ and Sadock VA. *Kaplan and Sadock's Synopsis of Psychiatry: Behavioral Sciences/clinical Psychiatry*, 10th edn. Lippincott Williams & Wilkins, 2007; p. 1072.

46. A. Mu (MOP) receptors are found in the brain in the cortex, thalamus, striosomes, and periaqueductal grey. The Mu1 subtype is responsible for supraspinal analgesia and physical dependence. The Mu 2 subtype is responsible for respiratory depression, euphoria, constipation, physical dependence, and miosis. Kappa (KOP) receptors are found in the hypothalamus, claustrum, and periaqueductal grey regions of the brain and the substantia gelatinosa of the spinal cord. They are involved in spinal analgesia, sedation, miosis, and inhibition of ADH release. Delta (DOP) receptors are seen in the brain in the regions of the pons, amygdala, olfactory bulbs, and the deep cortex. Their function includes analgesia, euphoria, and physical dependence. Sigma receptors, which mediate the antitussive action, are no longer considered to be opioid receptors. A new receptor called ORL1 has recently been identified, with an endogenous ligand called nociceptin. The ORL1 receptors do not bind opioid peptides or opiate drugs. This system is widely distributed in the brain and spinal cord. Its activation produces hyperalgesia in most instances. Many do not consider ORL1 as an opiate receptor. The International Union of Basic and Clinical Pharmacology has recently agreed to rename mu, kappa, and delta to MOP, KOP and DOP receptors respectively.

Corbett AD, Henderson G, McKnight AT, Paterson SJ. 75 years of opioid research: the exciting but vain quest for the Holy Grail. *British Journal of Pharmacology* 2006; **147**: S153–162.

47. C. Assessing the methadone dose equivalent of reported street heroin use is difficult because of the reliance on self-report and the variable purity of illicit heroin. Broadly speaking, 30–40 mL of 1 mg/mL mixture is approximately equivalent to 0.5 g of street heroin.

Gelder mg *et al.*, eds. *New Oxford Textbook of Psychiatry*. Oxford University Press, 2000, p. 527.

48. C. A controversial cannabis-related syndrome is amotivational syndrome. Whether the syndrome is related to cannabis use or reflects characterological traits in a subgroup of people regardless of cannabis use is under debate. Traditionally, amotivational syndrome has been associated with long-term heavy use and has been characterized by a person's unwillingness to persist in a task. Persons are described as becoming apathetic and anergic, and appearing indolent. Field studies of chronic heavy cannabis users in societies with a tradition of such use have not produced consistent evidence to demonstrate the existence of amotivational syndrome. Critics have questioned the methodological issues of the study. However, the possibility has been kept alive by reports that regular cannabis users experience a loss of ambition and impaired school and occupational performance.

Sadock BJ and Sadock VA. *Kaplan and Sadock's Synopsis of Psychiatry: Behavioral Sciences/clinical Psychiatry*, 10th edn. Lippincott Williams & Wilkins, 2007, p. 419.

49. C. Maternal smoking during pregnancy has been consistently associated with conduct disorder and delinquency and attention-deficit hyperactivity disorder (ADHD) in offspring during childhood and adolescence. This association has been found even after controlling for confounding variables such as socioeconomic status, maternal age, birth weight, and maternal psychopathology. This may be due to the effect of nicotine or may be genetically mediated. There may be other environmental risks that play a part in its development. More recent research has shown that the behavioural problems may not be a direct risk of smoking itself, but the presence of other genetic factors that may mediate the association between maternal smoking and conduct problems in children.

Button TM, Thapar A and McGuffin P. Relationship between antisocial behaviour, attention-deficit hyperactivity disorder and maternal prenatal smoking. *British Journal of Psychiatry* 2005; **187**: 155–160.

50. B. LSD and its metabolites are detectable in human urine for as long as 4 days after the ingestion of 0.2 mg of the drug. Amphetamines can be detected for 2–4 days; cocaine can be present for up to 3 days. Marijuana users may test positive in urine samples for up to 3 days after casual use; this can extend to up to 30 days for regular high-dose users.

Lowinson JH, Ruiz P, Millman RB and Langrod JG. *Substance Abuse: A Comprehensive Textbook*, 4th edn. Lippincott Williams & Wilkins, 2005, p. 572.

1. **A tumour in which of the following areas is most likely to lead to behavioural/psychiatric manifestation?**
   A. Frontal lobe
   B. Temporal lobe
   C. Posterior fossa
   D. Parietal lobe
   E. Occipital lobe

2. **Which of the following is least associated with a frontal lobe tumour?**
   A. Decline in IQ
   B. Dysexecutive syndrome
   C. Disinhibition
   D. Akinetic mutism
   E. Manic syndrome

3. **Factors affecting the presence of neuropsychiatric symptoms in head tumours include**
   A. Site of lesion
   B. Increased intracranial pressure
   C. Rapidity of growth
   D. Histopathology of the tumour
   E. All of the above

4. **Which of the following has been found to be effective in the treatment of pathological laughing and crying (PLAC) syndrome?**
   A. Valproate
   B. Moclobemide
   C. Citalopram
   D. Lithium
   E. Thyroxine

5. **The lifetime prevalence of psychosis in patients suffering from epilepsy is around**
   A. 1–2%
   B. 7–12%
   C. 16–22%
   D. 27–32%
   E. 37–42%

6. **Which of the following is the most important factor in increasing the risk of suicide in epilepsy?**
   A. Presence of comorbid psychiatric disorder
   B. Young male
   C. Temporal lobe seizure
   D. Greater duration of seizure disorder
   E. Inadequate therapy

7. **Andrew is a 30-year-old man who presented with frontal headaches and a history of complex partial seizures. Typically, his seizures begin with 20 seconds of orobuccal movements followed by 40 seconds of altered consciousness. At seizure onset, Andrew feels he must constantly think of the word 'Supercalifragilisticexpialidocious' and repeat this several times without him being able to control it. What is this phenomenon called?**
   A. Forced thinking
   B. Obsession
   C. Compulsion
   D. Forced normalization
   E. Periodic lateralization

8. **The phenomenon where the onset of peri-ictal psychosis occurs as a result of control of epileptic seizures is called**
   A. Forced normalization
   B. Forced thinking
   C. Periodic lateralization
   D. Twilight state
   E. Geschwind syndrome

9. **Which of the following is NOT considered a feature of irritable bowel syndrome (IBS)?**
   A. Abdominal discomfort not relieved by defaecation
   B. Altered stool frequency
   C. Altered stool form
   D. Altered stool passage
   E. Passage of mucus

10. **Which of the following is NOT a model that has been proposed to explain the relationship between IBS and high rates of psychiatric comorbidity?**
    A. Somatization disorder hypothesis
    B. Somatopsychic hypothesis
    C. Psychogenic hypothesis
    D. Self-selection hypothesis
    E. Conversion hypothesis

11. **Which of the following is a psychosocial risk factor for the development of peptic ulcer?**
    A. History of major depressive disorder
    B. History of an anxiety disorder
    C. History of sexual abuse
    D. History of childhood neglect
    E. All of the above

12. **Which of the following is NOT a risk factor for the development of peptic ulcer?**
    A. Cigarette smoking
    B. Heavy alcohol consumption
    C. Lack of sleep
    D. Not eating breakfast
    E. High socioeconomic status

13. **Which of the following is an early symptom/sign of HIV dementia?**
    A. Forgetfulness
    B. Confusion
    C. Disorientation
    D. Slowing of verbal responses
    E. Carphologia

14. **According to the WHO classification, the normal range of body mass index (BMI) is**
    A. 16–18.50
    B. 18.50–24.99
    C. 25–29.99
    D. 30–34.99
    E. None of the above

15. **Which of the following is considered the cardinal feature of delirium?**
    A. Disturbance of sleep wake cycle
    B. Psychomotor disturbance
    C. Hallucinations
    D. Disturbance of consciousness
    E. Affective lability

16. **Which of the following is a feature of systemic lupus erythematosus (SLE)?**

A. Late involvement of the central nervous system (CNS)

B. CNS events strongly correlate with systemic disease activity

C. Neuropsychiatric manifestations correlate with the presence of anticardiolipin antibodies

D. 90% of the people diagnosed with SLE suffer from depression

E. Stress has not been linked with exacerbation in SLE

17. **Which of the following is a *characteristic* feature of paediatric autoimmune neuropsychiatric disorder due to group A streptococcal infection (PANDAS)?**

A. Arthritis

B. Carditis

C. Rheumatic fever

D. Chorea

E. Tics

18. **Which of the following is the most common psychiatric manifestation of hyperthyroidism?**

A. Major depression

B. Anxiety disorder

C. Cognitive disorder

D. Psychosis

E. None of the above

19. **Which of the following is the most commonly reported psychiatric symptom in hypothyroidism?**

A. Depression

B. Cognitive disturbance

C. Anxiety

D. Psychosis

E. None of the above

20. **Regarding corticosteroid-induced neuropsychiatric complications, which of the following statements is true?**

A. Predominantly affective illness

B. Severity of symptoms is dose related

C. Complications tend to occur in the first 2 weeks of starting therapy

D. Lithium prophylaxis is helpful

E. All of the above

21. **Which of the following is the most common psychiatric manifestation of Cushing's syndrome?**

A. Major depression

B. Mania

C. Anxiety disorder

D. Psychosis

E. Cognitive disorders

22. **A 60-year-old woman who recently underwent radiation therapy to her neck presented with 'painful bones, renal stones, abdominal groans, and psychic moans'. Which of the following condition is she most likely to be suffering from?**

   A. Hyperparathyroidism
   B. Hypoparathyroidism
   C. Hyperthyroidism
   D. Hypothyroidism
   E. None of the above

23. **The prevalence of major depressive disorder in patients with Huntington's disease is around**

   A. 1%
   B. 5%
   C. 15%
   D. 40%
   E. 80%

24. **Which of the following is a feature of cognitive dysfunction in Huntington's disease?**

   A. Sparing of verbal recall
   B. Late-onset verbal memory and visuospatial dysfunction
   C. Sparing of procedural memory
   D. Early executive function loss
   E. Loss of speech comprehension before the loss of speech production

25. **Which of the following is a feature of amnestic mild cognitive impairment (MCI)?**

   A. Absence of subjective memory complaints
   B. Absence of memory impairment relative to age-matched healthy control
   C. Presence of evidence of clinical dementia
   D. Presence of difficulties in ADL
   E. Amyloid deposits and tau-positive tangles are seen more often in the mesial temporal lobes than in normal controls

26. **Which of the following is a monogenic ischaemic stroke syndrome?**

   A. CADASIL
   B. Moya Moya disease
   C. Reversible posterior leucoencephalopathy
   D. Binswanger's disease
   E. Necrotizing arteritis

27. Which of the following is NOT a feature of Stage I Alzheimer's dementia?

A. Memory impairment
B. Visuospatial impairment
C. Anomia
D. Impairment in calculation
E. Background slowing on EEG

28. Which of the following is NOT a feature of Binswanger's disease?

A. Rapidly progressive dementia
B. Clinical signs may include parkinsonian syndrome
C. Fluctuating mental state is seen
D. Deep white mater demyelination in periventricular areas
E. Typically seen in chronic hypertensive patients

29. Which of the following is true regarding frontotemporal dementia (FTD)?

A. Semantic dementia is the most common subtype
B. The frontal variant is characterized by loss of word meaning and object recognition
C. 40% of cases of FTD are familial autosomal dominant
D. Pick bodies are immunoreactive to ubiquitin, but not to tau
E. Pick's disease is the most common histological variant

30. HIV-induced cognitive deficits have been proposed to be due to

A. Increased calcium-induced cell injury
B. Altered brain glucose metabolism
C. TNF-alpha-induced apoptosis
D. NMDA-related excitotoxicity
E. All of the above

31. Which of the following is the most common intracranial opportunistic infection in HIV?

A. Toxoplasmosis
B. Cryptococcosis
C. Cytomegalovirus (CMV) infection
D. Herpes simplex virus (HSV)
E. Progressive multifocal leucoencephalitis

32. All of the following features of hyperactive delirium help differentiate it from hypoactive delirium, except

A. Restlessness
B. Hallucinations
C. Fast EEG activity
D. Better prognosis
E. Increased speech

33. **All of the following factors render a person at high risk for development of post-operative delirium except**
    A. Baseline cognitive deficit
    B. Old age
    C. Multiple medication
    D. Emergency procedures
    E. High albumin

34. **Which of the following medication used in elderly people has the least propensity to induce delirium?**
    A. Digoxin
    B. Prednisolone
    C. Nifedipine
    D. Cimetidine
    E. Atenolol

35. **All of the following are causes of diffuse slowing on EEG except**
    A. Alcohol withdrawal delirium
    B. Post-traumatic delirium
    C. Anticholinergic delirium
    D. Hepatic encephalopathy delirium
    E. Hypoxic delirium

36. **In children with PANDAS, which symptoms are least common?**
    A. Obsessions
    B. Emotional lability
    C. Tics
    D. Separation anxiety
    E. Auditory hallucinations

37. **Which is the most common site for the primary tumour in a metastatic brain cancer?**
    A. Lung
    B. Breast
    C. Kidney
    D. Gastrointestinal tract (GIT)
    E. Prostate

38. **A 40-year-old lady with multiple sclerosis (MS) was diagnosed with depression. She is on a number of medications for her MS. Of the following medication she is on, which is most likely to be associated with depressive symptoms?**
    A. Gabapentin
    B. Amantadine
    C. Baclofen
    D. Interferon 1-beta
    E. None of the above

39. John is a 30-year-old man being treated for psychotic depression with selective serotonin uptake inhibitors (SSRIs) and antipsychotics. He takes an overdose of his medications and is admitted to the medical unit with features of tremor and hyperthermia. He does not know which medications he has taken. Which of the following points to a diagnosis of serotonin syndrome rather than neuroleptic malignant syndrome?

    A. Myoclonus
    B. 'Lead-pipe' muscle rigidity
    C. Rhabdomyolysis
    D. Elevated creatine phosphokinase (CPK)
    E. Delirium

40. James was admitted to the medical unit following an attempt of deliberate self-harm (DSH). What percentage of people completes suicide within a year of the DSH attempt?

    A. 1%
    B. 10%
    C. 20%
    D. 30%
    E. 40%

41. Which is the antipsychotic of choice for a 75-year-old man with Parkinson's disease who presented with psychotic symptoms?

    A. Aripiprazole
    B. Risperidone
    C. Olanzapine
    D. Quetiapine
    E. Haloperidol

42. If a patient continues to take sodium valproate throughout her pregnancy what is the risk of the baby having a neural tube defect?

    A. 0.05–0.1%
    B. 1–2%
    C. 10–20%
    D. 20–30%
    E. 30–40%

43. Which of the following is NOT a feature of chronic fatigue syndrome (CFS)?

    A. Late insomnia
    B. Severe unexplained fatigue not resolved by rest
    C. Duration more than 6 months
    D. Post-exertional malaise
    E. Muscle aches and pains

44. **Which antidepressant has got good evidence for its use in post-myocardial infarction depression?**
    A. Fluoxetine
    B. Citalopram
    C. Reboxetine
    D. Mirtazapine
    E. Sertraline

45. **Which of the following is the treatment of choice for premenstrual dysphoric disorder?**
    A. SSRI
    B. Primrose oil
    C. Vitamin E
    D. Vitamin A
    E. St John's Wort

46. **Mothers with anorexia nervosa are at high risk for having babies with**
    A. Greater congenital malformations
    B. Larger birth weight
    C. Are born post term
    D. Macrocephaly
    E. Lower birth weight

47. **The percentage of people with mental illness who were in contact with psychiatric services within 1 week of suicide is**
    A. 10%
    B. 20%
    C. 30%
    D. 40%
    E. 50%

48. **Which of the following is the best screening tool used in post-natal depression?**
    A. Hamilton depression rating scale
    B. Edinburgh postnatal depression scale
    C. Montgomery Asberg depression rating scale
    D. Hospital anxiety and depression scale
    E. Beck's depression inventory

49. **Which of the following is least associated with suicide?**
    A. Depression
    B. Mania
    C. Schizophrenia
    D. Anxiety disorder
    E. Dementia

50. Maria suffered from postpartum blues during the immediate postpartum period, what is the chance that she develops postpartum depression?

    A. 1–5%
    B. 10–15%
    C. 20–25%
    D. 30–35%
    E. 40–45%

1. A. Frontal lobe tumours have been reported to be associated with psychiatric and behavioural symptoms in as much as 90% of cases. Frontal lobe tumours are associated with symptoms suggestive of mood disturbances and psychoses, including mania and hypomania, depression, catatonia, delusions, and hallucinations. Temporal lobe tumours cause psychiatric and behavioural symptoms in as much as 50–55% of the cases. Pituitary tumours cause psychiatric manifestations in as many as 60% of cases; parietal lobe – 15%; occipital lobe – 25%; and diencephalic tumours – 50%.

Kaplan HI. *Kaplan and Sadock's Comprehensive Textbook of Psychiatry*, 8th edn. Lippincott Williams and Wilkins, 2004, p. 363.

2. A. Frontal lobe tumours do not generally cause a decline in IQ. Tumours of the frontal lobes tend to produce symptoms that reflect their anatomical locations. They usually interfere with frontally mediated executive functions. Tumours involving the anterior cingulate are associated with akinetic mutism. Tumours involving the dorsolateral prefrontal convexities are typically associated with apathy, abulia, lack of spontaneity, psychomotor retardation, reduced ability to plan ahead, motor impersistence, and impaired attention and concentration. Patients with orbitofrontal tumours often exhibit personality changes, irritability and mood lability, behavioural disinhibition and impulsivity, lack of insight, and poor judgement. Tumours of the ventral right frontal lobe are often associated with euphoria. Tumours of the left frontal lobe often cause decreased speech fluency and diminished verbal output, word-finding problems, and circumlocutory speech, whereas tumours affecting both frontal lobes are often associated with confabulation, Capgras' syndrome, or reduplicative paramnesias, or a combination of these.

Kaplan HI. *Kaplan and Sadock's Comprehensive Textbook of Psychiatry*, 8th edn. Lippincott Williams and Wilkins, 2004, p. 363.

3. E. The anatomical location of a tumour is an important factor that predicts the development of neuropsychiatric problems in the population. For example, left temporal lobe tumours are most commonly associated with psychosis. To some extent, the symptoms represent the underlying function of the involved lobe. The aggressiveness of the tumour itself and the rapidity and extent of its spread are also believed to be important factors in the type, acuity, and severity of psychiatric and behavioural symptoms that may be associated with it. Thus, rapidly growing tumours are frequently associated with more acute psychiatric symptomatology, as well as significant neurocognitive impairment. In this case, raised intracranial tension is associated with rapid growth and hence more behavioural problems. In general, the specific histological characteristics of brain tumours have not been shown to be correlated with specific psychiatric and behavioural symptoms. However, as noted previously, more aggressive tumours, such as high-grade gliomas, are more likely to be associated with acute psychiatric and behavioural symptoms than are slower growing malignant and benign tumours.

Kaplan HI. *Kaplan and Sadock's Comprehensive Textbook of Psychiatry*, 8th ed. Lippincott Williams and Wilkins, 2004, p. 363.

4. C. Pathological emotions are characterized by episodes of laughing or crying, or both, that are not appropriate to the context. They may be spontaneous or triggered by non-emotional events. Pathological emotions have classically been explained as secondary to the bilateral interruption of descending neocortical upper motor neuron innervations of bulbar motor nuclei. Some patients with pathological emotions have bilateral lesions and pseudobulbar palsy, but others do not. Most recently, the frontopontocerebellar pathways have been implicated in the pathogenesis of pathological emotions. It is seen in about 15% of patients with stroke. Citalopram, as well as nortriptyline, have been found to be effective in the treatment of pathological crying after stroke in randomized placebo-controlled trials. In addition, post-stroke depression and PLAC appear to be independent phenomena, although they may coexist.

Kaplan HI. *Kaplan and Sadock's Comprehensive Textbook of Psychiatry*, 8th edn. Lippincott Williams and Wilkins, 2004, p. 361.

5. B. Psychosis is the specific psychiatric disorder most clearly associated with epilepsy. The lifelong prevalence of all psychotic disorders among epileptic patients ranges from 7% to 12%. Patients whose epilepsy has a mediobasal temporal focus are especially at risk. Studies on the laterality of the seizure focus suggest an association of a left-sided focus with psychosis. Although conclusions derived from surface EEG recording are open to criticism, depth recordings of presurgical patients show that twice as many patients with left temporal lesions have psychosis.

Kaplan HI. *Kaplan and Sadock's Comprehensive Textbook of Psychiatry*, 8th edn. Lippincott Williams and Wilkins, 2004, p. 379.

6. A. Suicide is increased fivefold among patients with epilepsy. Among patients presenting with self-harm, epileptic subjects are over-represented from five- to sevenfold. Risk factors for suicide in epilepsy are ranked as follows: (1) Comorbid psychiatric disorders (2) relatively young males (ages 25–49 years); (3) temporal lobe seizures (with brain lesions); (4) prolonged duration of the seizure disorder (5) inadequate therapy (6) personal, social, or occupational difficulties; and (7) availability of large amounts of antiepileptic drugs.

Trimble M and Schmitz B. *The Neuropsychiatry of Epilepsy*. Cambridge University Press, 2002, p. 108.

7. A. This type of psychic aura is called 'forced thinking,' characterized by recurrent intrusive thoughts, ideas, or crowding of thoughts. Forced thinking must be distinguished from obsessional thoughts and compulsive urges. Epileptic patients with forced thinking experience their thoughts as stereotypical, out-of-context, brief, and irrational, but not necessarily as ego dystonic. Periodic lateralizations are recurrent EEG complexes that may be associated with prolonged confusional behaviour and focal cognitive changes.

Kaplan HI. *Kaplan and Sadock's Comprehensive Textbook of Psychiatry*, 8th edn. Lippincott Williams and Wilkins, 2004; p. 381.

8. A. Periictal psychotic symptoms more often worsen with increasing seizure activity. Rarely, psychotic symptoms alternate with seizure activity. In this 'alternating psychosis', as long as the patient's seizures are not controlled, they are free of psychotic symptoms, but when they are seizure free and their EEG has 'forced' or 'paradoxical normalization', they manifest psychotic symptoms. This alternating pattern is much less common than the increased emergence of psychotic behaviour with increasing seizure activity. Twilight states are episodes of confusion that may be associated with the seizure (ictal) or after a seizure (post ictal). They may be associated with odd behaviours, and the patient is usually not conscious about the behaviour. Geschwind syndrome is otherwise called epileptic personality. It consists of a cluster of personality traits including hyposexuality, hypergraphia, hyperviscosity, hyperreligiosity seen in patients with long-standing epilepsy.

Kaplan HI. *Kaplan and Sadock's Comprehensive Textbook of Psychiatry*, 8th edn. Lippincott Williams and Wilkins, 2004 p. 382.

9. A. IBS is the prototypical functional gastrointestinal disorder characterized by abdominal pain and diarrhoea or constipation. The International Congress of Gastroenterology has developed a standardized set of criteria for IBS. They include either abdominal pain relieved by defaecation or associated with a change in frequency or consistency of stool; or disturbed defaecation involving two or more of the following: altered stool frequency; altered stool form hard or loose and watery; altered stool passage straining or urgency or feeling of incomplete evacuation; passage of mucus. IBS can be categorized into diarrhoea-predominant, constipation-predominant, and mixed subtypes. Medical treatment often targets the predominant symptom. IBS accounts for as much as 50% of all outpatient evaluations done by gastroenterologists.

Kaplan HI. *Kaplan and Sadock's Comprehensive Textbook of Psychiatry*, 8th edn. Lippincott Williams and Wilkins, 2004 p. 2115.

10. E. Studies of psychiatric comorbidity in IBS estimate rates of comorbidity at 42–64% of all IBS patients. The exact mechanism for high rates of psychiatric comorbidity in IBS is unknown. Four models have been proposed to explain the relationship between IBS and high rates of psychiatric comorbidity. The first model is the somatization disorder hypothesis. This model classifies IBS as one of a group of diagnoses that can be made from a primary somatization disorder or other somatoform disorder. The somatopsychic hypothesis states that psychological symptoms are the result of chronic gastrointestinal distress and the unsatisfactory interaction with healthcare providers who do not accurately diagnose and treat IBS. Psychogenic hypothesis states that specific psychiatric disorders cause IBS for a significant proportion of patients. Panic disorder, in particular, is proposed as a cause for secondary IBS. The self-selection model proposes that psychiatric comorbidity increases the rate of treatment seeking in patients who have IBS.

Kaplan HI. *Kaplan and Sadock's Comprehensive Textbook of Psychiatry*, 8th edn. Lippincott Williams and Wilkins, 2004 p. 2118.

11. E. Since the discovery of *Helicobacter pylori*, interest in the association of peptic ulcer and psychosocial factors has diminished. Nevertheless, psychosocial factors do play a role in the development of ulcers in susceptible individuals. Data from the National Comorbidity Survey have shown that generalized anxiety disorder (GAD) is associated with an increased risk of self-reported peptic ulcer disease. Longitudinal prospective studies have shown that depression and anxiety at baseline increase the risk of ulcer development. Childhood physical abuse, sexual abuse, and neglect are also associated with a statistically increased risk of peptic ulceration in addition to other physical conditions. Acute severe stress in human beings, provoked by wars or earthquakes, can precipitate ulceration in susceptible individuals. Once formed, psychosocial factors can delay recovery and contribute to a worse prognosis.

Lloyd G and Guthrie E. *Handbook of Liaison Psychiatry*, illustrated edition. Cambridge University Press, 2007, p. 392.

12. E. Lifestyle factors predict the development of peptic ulcer in susceptible individuals. They are potential mediators in the aetiological matrix between stress and ulcer. These include cigarette smoking; heavy alcohol consumption; lack of sleep; not eating breakfast; non-steroidal anti-inflammatory drugs; hard on-the-job labour and low socioeconomic status.

Lloyd G and Guthrie E. *Handbook of Liaison Psychiatry*, illustrated edition. Cambridge University Press, 2007. p. 392.

13. A. Organic and neuropsychiatric disorders in HIV are common, and may result from the direct effects of HIV, opportunistic infections, effects of neoplasms, metabolic abnormalities, iatrogenic interventions and others. The prevalence of HIV dementia is around 10–15%. Cognitive changes may be directly due to the effects of HIV itself, secondary to opportunistic infection following treatment, or due to pre-existing psychological morbidity. These changes may be classified into early and late. Early symptoms consist of forgetfulness, poor concentration, balance problems, apathy, withdrawal, dysphoric mood, and dyspraxia. Symptoms that are suggestive of a late change include disorientation, confusion, peripheral neuropathies, slowed verbal responses, indifference to illness, organic psychosis, incontinence, and carphologia (picking imaginary objects and bed linen).

Lloyd G and Guthrie E. *Handbook of Liaison Psychiatry*, illustrated edition. Cambridge University Press, 2007, p. 482.

14. B. BMI is a simple index of weight-for-height that is commonly used to classify underweight, overweight, and obesity in adults. It is defined as the weight in kilograms divided by the square of the height in metres (kg/m^2). BMI values are age independent and the same for both sexes. However, BMI may not correspond to the same degree of fatness in different populations due, in part, to different body proportions. The health risks associated with increasing BMI are continuous and the interpretation of BMI grading in relation to risk may differ for different populations: underweight <18.50; normal range 18.50–24.99; overweight ≥25.00; pre-obese 25.00–29.99; obese ≥30.00; obese class I 30.00–34.99; obese class II 35.00–39.99; obese class III ≥40.00.

World Health Organization. *Obesity: Preventing and Managing the Global* Epidemic. Report of a WHO Consultation. WHO Technical Report Series 894. Geneva, 2000.

15. D. The clinical presentation of delirium is defined by psychopathology and temporal course. It is usually of acute onset and the cardinal feature is a disturbance in consciousness. Impairment of consciousness is the key feature that separates delirium from most other psychiatric disorders. There is a continuum between mild impairment of consciousness and near unconsciousness. There is fluctuation in intensity, and symptoms are often worse at night. The other features are an inability to focus and maintain attention, perceptual disturbances, disorientation in time and/or space, rarely to people (though false recognition is common) and almost never to self. Disorientation to time is often the first warning sign of delirium. Attention is poor and the patient is easily distractable, looking either apathetic or intensely focused upon something. Psychomotor disturbance may be in the form of agitation or retardation. Other features may include lability of mood and incoherent speech.

Gelder M, Harrison P, and Cowen P. *Shorter Oxford Textbook of Psychiatry*, 5th edn. Oxford University Press, 2006; p. 329.

16. C. Psychiatric manifestations are common in SLE. Up to 90% of patients have some neuropsychiatric manifestation. In most patients, CNS complications present early in the illness, and studies that have looked into it have found no relationship between systemic disease activity and neuropsychiatric manifestations. In fact, neuropsychiatric causes are second only to renal causes as far as mortality is concerned in these patients. These complications include stroke, seizures, transverse myelitis, etc. Cognitive deficits are the most common neuropsychiatric manifestation in these patients. It is present in up to 80% of the patient sample. These have been correlated with the presence of anticardiolipin antibody. In this way, most psychiatric illnesses have been correlated with the presence of an antibody in the blood. Depression has been reported in up to 40% of people with SLE. Psychiatric symptoms in SLE have been attributed to direct CNS involvement, infections, side-effects of medications, reactions to chronic illness and primary psychiatric illness. Similarly, stress has been linked to exacerbation of SLE. This is said to be mediated through the immune system.

Levenson JL. *Essentials of Psychosomatic Medicine*, 1st edn. American Psychiatric Press, 2006, 139–141.

Stojanovicha L, Zandman-Goddardb G, Pavlovicha S and Sikanichd N. Psychiatric manifestations in systemic lupus erythematosus *Autoimmunity Reviews* 2007; **66**: 421–426.

17. E. PANDAS is a controversial disease. In fact, Levinson says that it is not a diagnosis, but a syndrome where obsessive compulsive disorder and tics have been exacerbated in children following a group A beta-haemolytic streptococcal (GABHS) infection. The diagnostic criteria for PANDAS that were proposed by Swedo *et al.* in 1998 include the following: OCD and/or chronic tic disorder (Tourette's, chronic motor, or vocal tic disorder) that meets the DSM-IV diagnostic criteria; age at onset between 3 years and the onset of puberty; clinical course with an abrupt onset of symptoms and/or a pattern of dramatic recurrent exacerbations and remissions; temporal relation between GABHS infection and onset and/or exacerbations of clinical symptoms; and neurologic abnormalities such as motoric hyperactivity, tics, or choreiform activity during an exacerbation.

James L. *Levenson Essentials of Psychosomatic Medicine*, 1st edn. American Psychiatric Press, 2006, p. 181.

Swedo SE, Leonard HL, Garvey M, *et al.* Pediatric autoimmune neuropsychiatric disorders associated with streptococcal infections: clinical description of the first 50 cases. *American Journal of Psychiatry* 1998; **155**: 264–271.

18. A. Despite the fact that anxiety is a cardinal feature of hyperthyroidism, anxiety disorders are observed in only up to 15% of the patients. Major depression is the most common psychiatric manifestation, seen in up to 25% of the people diagnosed with hyperthyroidism. Cognitive disturbance is seen in around 7.5% of patients. Mania and hypomania are less common, with a prevalence of around 2%, and psychosis occurs in around 2% of the population with hyperthyroidism.

Hales RE and Yudofsky SC. *The American Psychiatric Publishing Textbook of Neuropsychiatry and Clinical Neurosciences*, 4th edn. American Psychiatric Press, 2002, pp. 858–860.

19. B. Patients with hypothyroidism present with all of the above symptoms. But the most commonly reported psychiatric symptoms are that of cognition, which occurs in around 45% of the patients. This can extend from mild subjective slowing to delirious and even encephalopathic states. Delirium is the most severe manifestation of hypothyroidism. Depression is the second most frequent psychiatric syndrome. Anxiety disorder is present in around 30% of the patients, and although myxoedema madness 'psychosis' is one of the most common symptoms reported in the literature, it represents only around 5% of psychiatric morbidity in these patients.

Hales RE and Yudofsky S.C. *The American Psychiatric Publishing Textbook of Neuropsychiatry and Clinical Neurosciences*, 4th edn. 2002, p. 856–857.

20. E. Nearly all steroids have been implicated. Psychiatric symptoms are mostly affective in nature, more specifically elation. Psychosis, delirium, and anxiety have been reported. Steroid-induced psychosis may be secondary to delirium, an exacerbation of pre-existing psychosis or frank psychosis precipitated by steroids (this includes mania). The prevalence of psychiatric disturbance in patients who have been administered corticosteroids is said to be dose related. Various strategies to prevent the onset of steroid-induced psychiatric manifestations include administering the medication in divided doses, enteric coated preparations, lithium, and valproate prophylaxis for those with a previous history. Tricyclic antidepressants (TCAs) are best avoided as these have been associated with an exacerbation of symptoms.

Hales RE and Yudofsky SC. *The American Psychiatric Publishing Textbook of Neuropsychiatry and Clinical Neurosciences*, 4th edn. American Psychiatric Press 2002, p. 863.

21. A. Full depressive syndrome has been reported in up to 70% of people with Cushing's syndrome. The most common cause of Cushing's syndrome is pharmacological. Cushing's disease is a primary pituitary tumour, which secretes an excess of adrenocorticotropic hormone (ACTH). Psychiatric manifestations may be due to the direct effects of elevated corticosteroids on the neurons or due to hypothalamic dysfunction. The neocortex and hippocampus have glucocorticoid receptors, the action on which could explain the cognitive and mood disorder seen in these patients. Cushing's disease has been associated with a reduction in hippocampal volume, which is reversed on correction of steroid levels. There is also some evidence to show that stress could be associated with exacerbation of the illness.

Levenson JL. *Essentials of Psychosomatic Medicine*, 1st edn. American Psychiatric Press, 2006, p. 96.

22. A. This patient shows the classical features of hyperparathyroidism leading to hypercalcaemia, possibly precipitated by the irradiation to the neck. The psychic moans are most commonly due to depression and cognitive symptoms. These have been correlated with the degree of calcium elevation. In severe cases, confusion, catatonia, agitation, psychosis, and coma can occur. Most patients improve with treatment and correction of calcium levels.

Hales RE and Yudofsky SC. *The American Psychiatric Publishing Textbook of Neuropsychiatry and Clinical Neurosciences*, 4th edn. American Psychiatric Press 2002, p. 867.

23. D.   Huntington's disease is an autosomal dominant disorder resulting from a mutation on chromosome 4, which leads to an increased number of CAG trinucleotide repeats from 6–34 to 39–86. Patients with longer trinucleotide repeat lengths have an earlier age of onset and more rapid progression than those with fewer repeats. It is seen that those who inherit the disease from the paternal side have a greater number of repeats and hence show an earlier age of onset, a phenomenon called genetic anticipation. Clinically, Huntington's disease is manifested by the triad of chorea, dementia, and psychiatric symptoms. Approximately 40% of patients exhibit major depressive disorders or meet criteria for dysthymia. Approximately 10% of patients exhibit hypomania and a few may have manic episodes. Apathy, irritability, and disinhibition may be present independent of a mood disorder. Sexual misconduct is more common, occurring in up to 20% of Huntington's disease patients. The rate of suicide is increased up to four times in patients with Huntington's disease. Psychiatric symptoms do not correlate with the CAG repeat length.

Cummings JL. Mega M.S. *Neuropsychiatry and Behavioural Neuroscience*, 2nd edn. Oxford University Press, 2003, p. 272.

24. D.   Verbal recognition is relatively spared compared with recall, which suggests a retrieval problem rather than an encoding problem. Problems with verbal memory and visuospatial function appear early in Huntington's disease, but don't progress as much as in patients with Alzheimer's. The picture is typical of a subcortical dementia involving frontal subcortical circuits. Patients with Huntington's disease show a typical loss of procedural memory. Executive function is lost early in the disease. They also show psychomotor slowing and attentional deficits that correlate with activities of daily living (ADL). Unlike psychiatric symptoms, cognitive symptoms correlate with the number of trinucleotide repeats. Speech comprehension is maintained late into the disease well after intelligible speech production is lost.

Cummings JL and Mega MS. *Neuropsychiatry and Behavioural Neuroscience*, 2nd edn. Oxford University Press 2003, p. 272.

25. E.   MCI is a syndrome characterized by the presence of cognitive decline greater than that expected for age and education level along with normal ADL. It is, thus, distinct from dementia, in which cognitive deficits are more severe and widespread and have a significant effect on daily function. A further subtype of MCI, amnestic subtype, has a higher rate of conversion to Alzheimer's disease. They characterized by memory complaints, corroborated by an informant: the presence of memory impairment relative to age- and education-matched healthy people; typical general cognitive function; largely intact ADL; and not clinically demented. Prevalence in population-based epidemiological studies ranges from 3% to 19% in adults older than 65 years. Compared with people with dementia and normal controls, individuals with MCI have intermediate amounts of Alzheimer's disease pathology, including amyloid deposition and tau-positive tangles in the mesial temporal lobes.

Gauthier S, Reisberg B, Zaudig M, *et al*. Mild cognitive impairment. *Lancet* **367**: 1262–1270.

26. A.   CADASIL (cerebral autosomal dominant arteriopathy with subcortical infarcts and leucoencephalopathy) is an autosomal dominant familial trait linked in several families to a mutation in the Notch 3 gene on chromosome 19. It presents as recurrent small-vessel strokes, beginning in early adulthood, leading to extensive symmetric white matter changes similar to Binswanger's disease and progressive dementia. The genetic nature of the syndrome may not be fully apparent because of the low penetrance. Approximately 40% of patients have migraine with aura. CADASIL is the only monogenic ischaemic stroke syndrome described. Genetic testing is available.

Kasper DL, *et al*. *Harrison's Principles of Internal Medicine*. McGraw-Hill, 2005.

27. E. According to Cummings, Alzheimer's disease progresses through three stages. In the first stage, the patient has anomia, defective visuospatial skills and calculation ability along with an indifferent personality. Examination of the motor system and EEG may be relatively normal, although some medial temporal atrophy may be noted in a structural brain scan. In the second stage of dementia, the patient has fluent aphasia and further deterioration in memory, visuospatial skills, and personality. In addition, there may be motor restlessness on examination. EEG may show background slowing and a structural brain scan may show temperoparietal atrophy. In the third and final stage, there is severe impairment in intellectual function and speech disturbances characterized by palilalia, echolalia, or mutism. In addition, there is sphincter disturbances, diffuse slowing on EEG and diffuse atrophy on structural scan.

Cummings JL and Mega MS. *Neuropsychiatry and Behavioural Neuroscience*, 2nd edn. Oxford University Press, 2003, p. 148.

28. A. Binswanger's disease is a slowly progressive dementia associated with subacute progression of focal neurological deficits in chronically hypertensive patients. These deficits could involve pseudobulbar, pyramidal, and parkinsonian features. Incontinence and fluctuating cognition may be seen. The periventricular area shows white matter demyelination, especially resulting from diffuse ischaemic damage. Lacunar infarcts are frequently absent. In patients thought to have multi-infarct dementia, leucoaraiosis is found in at least three quarters.

Stein G and Wilkinson G. *Seminars in General Adult Psychiatry*, 2nd edn. RCPsych Publications, 2007, p. 516.

29. C. Forty per cent of cases of FTD are familial, mainly autosomal dominant. Mutations in the tau gene were first found in FTD with parkinsonism linked to chromosome 17 (FTDP-17). Histologically FTD consist of five types. The motor neuron type with inclusions reactive for ubiquitin but not for tau is the most frequent type. The second most common is a corticobasal degeneration type that is tau positive but with ubiquitin-negative inclusions. The third is Pick's disease with neuronal loss, widespread gliosis, and inflated neurons with inclusions positive for both tau and ubiquitin. The familial pattern has tau-positive inclusions in neurons and glial cells. Clinically frontal lobe variant accounts for the most common presentation (70%). They present with symptoms suggestive of frontal lobe dysfunction. Temporal variants are of two types: semantic and progressive aphasic. Semantic dementia accounts for about 15% of the presentation. They show progressive loss of word meaning and object or face identity. Ten per cent of cases are of the progressive aphasic type.

Stein G and Wilkinson G. *Seminars in General Adult Psychiatry*, 2nd edn. RCPsych Publications, 2007, p. 519.

Cummings JL and Mega MS. *Neuropsychiatry and Behavioural Neuroscience*, 2nd edn. Oxford University Press, 2003. p. 150.

30. E. All of the given mechanisms have been proposed to be the aetiopathogenesis behind cognitive deficits in HIV infection. In the process of binding to a CD4+ receptor-containing cells, HIV gp120 binds to a calcium channel and increases intracellular free calcium. This also leads to an alteration in glucose metabolism, leading to brain dysfunction. Further, the viral genome is incorporated into the host genome, which leads to the release of more injurious compounds. These include substances such as quinolinic acid, superoxide anions, and other proinflammatory cytokines. These products, especially quinolinic acid, act as NMDA agonists, leading to excitotoxicity and cell death. TNF-alpha, one of the proinflammatory cytokines, is also known to trigger apoptosis or programmed cell death.

Hales RE and Yudofsky SC. *The American Psychiatric Publishing Textbook of Neuropsychiatry and Clinical Neurosciences*, 4th edn. American Psychiatric Press, 2002, p. 786.

31. A. Toxoplasmosis is the most common opportunistic infection seen in AIDS patients. They may present with focal or diffuse cognitive or affective symptoms. Imaging may help with the diagnosis but may be normal in many cases. Definitive diagnosis is by biopsy. Cryptococcosis presents as meningitis with headache and fever. Other viral infections of the brain may present with personality and behavioural changes. HSV encephalitis typically presents with temporal lobe symptoms. CMV infection presents as encephalitis, retinitis, and peripheral neuropathies with demyelination. Progressive multifocal leucoencephalopathy is caused by a papova virus. The prognosis is poor.

Hales RE and Yudofsky SC. *The American Psychiatric Publishing Textbook of Neuropsychiatry and Clinical Neurosciences*, 4th edn. American Psychiatric Press, 2002, p. 787.

32. C. Hyperactive delirium is characterized by increased activity levels, including restlessness, loss of control of activities, and increased speed of action. Hypoactive delirium on the other hand is characterized by decreased activity levels including apathy, listlessness, and decreased speed of action. Hyperactive delirium may present with pressure of speech, altered content, and aggression, whereas hypoactive delirium usually presents with a decreased amount of speech and hypersomnolence. Hyperactive delirium is said to have a better prognosis than hypoactive delirium. But both types of delirium are characterized by diffuse slowing on the EEG.

Hales RE and Yudofsky SC. *The American Psychiatric Publishing Textbook of Neuropsychiatry and Clinical Neurosciences*, 4th edn. American Psychiatric Press 2002, p. 543.

33. E. Along with a number of other factors, including extremes of age, pre-existing cognitive impairment, central nervous system disorders, medical comorbidity, medications, hypothermia, and electrolyte imbalance, hypoalbuminaemia is an important often unnoticed risk factor. Hypoalbuminaemia results in greater bioavailability of many drugs that use albumin as a transporter protein. This leads to greater side-effects resulting in delirium. This may not be picked up by carrying out therapeutic drug monitoring. In addition to the above, a number of surgical factors predispose to delirium, including long duration of operation, emergency procedures, and type of surgery (e.g. hip surgery).

Hales RE and Yudofsky SC. *The American Psychiatric Publishing Textbook of Neuropsychiatry and Clinical Neurosciences*, 4th edn. American Psychiatric Press, 2002, p. 534.

34. E. Atenolol is a water-soluble selective beta-blocker which has almost nil anticholinergic action. Further, due to its water-soluble property, atenolol does not cross the blood–brain barrier. All the other medications have some anticholinergic properties and may contribute to the presence of delirium, especially in older patients, who are more vulnerable and are often using multiple medications. Of these, cimetidine and prednisolone are particularly important.

Hales RE and Yudofsky SC. *The American Psychiatric Publishing Textbook of Neuropsychiatry and Clinical Neurosciences*, 4th edn. American Psychiatric Press, 2002, p. 535.

35. A. Alcohol withdrawal delirium and benzodiazepine intoxication delirium present with low-voltage fast-activity on EEG. All the other options present with diffuse slowing, which is the pattern seen in most other cases. Frontocentral spikes are usually seen in toxic delirium, i.e. usually due to hypnosedative withdrawal or TCA and phenothiazine intoxication. Epileptiform activity may suggest post-ictal states or non-convulsive status epilepticus.

Hales RE and Yudofsky SC. *The American Psychiatric Publishing Textbook of Neuropsychiatry and Clinical Neurosciences*, 4th edn. American Psychiatric Press, 2002, p. 539.

36. E.   Motoric hyperactivity, impulsivity, night-time difficulties, distractibility and inattention, emotional lability, some degree of anorexia, and separation anxiety are some of the behavioural symptoms reported in association with PANDAS. From the choices available, it appears auditory hallucinations would be the least common symptom. Two antibodies have been found to be suggestive of PANDAS, D8/17 and-anti basal ganglia antibody. Both are not specific for PANDAS. Rising antistreptolysin O (ASO) or anti-DNAse B titres are suggestive of recent GABHS infection.

Schneider R, Robinson. M and Levenson J. Psychiatry in the medically ill. *Psychiatric Clinics of North America* 2002, **25**: 9.

37. A.   Of patients with intracerebral metastases, 40% originate in the lung, 20% are from breast tumours, 10% are melanomas, 7% arise from the genitourinary tract, 7% from the GIT, and 5% are of gynaecological origin.

Cummings JL and Mega MS. *Neuropsychiatry and Behavioural Neuroscience*, 2nd edn. Oxford University Press 2003, p. 402.

38. D.   All of the present neuromedical treatments for MS including, corticosteroids, beta-interferons, glatiramer acetate, and immunosuppressants, are suspected to affect mood, at least in some individuals. Corticosteroids are associated with euphoria initially and long-term intake could lead to a depressive state. Initial studies of interferon beta-1b, an immunomodulatory cytokine used to reduce MS disease activity over prolonged periods, found increases in depression following initiation of treatment, and increased risk of suicide attempts. More recent studies have shown that this association may not be as robust as it was thought before. In fact, at least one study has shown that baseline depression levels actually drop following treatment with the medication. It is now thought that baseline or previous history of depression is more likely to predict the development of depressive symptoms during treatment. The BNF has a warning note asking clinicians to avoid the prescription of interferon beta in patients who have a history of severe depression and suicidal ideation. Depression is also a side-effect of Baclofen, but the association is less than with interferon beta.

Feinstein A, O'Connor P and Feinstein K. Multiple Sclerosis, interferon beta-1b and depression. *Journal of Neurology* 2002; **249**: 815–820.

Goldman Consensus Group. The Goldman consensus statement on depression in multiple sclerosis. *Multiple Sclerosis* 2005; **11**: 328–337.

39. A.   Neuroleptic malignant syndrome occurs in the setting of antipsychotic use or the sudden withdrawal of dopaminergic drugs and is characterized by 'lead-pipe' muscle rigidity, extrapyramidal side-effects, autonomic dysregulation, and hyperthermia. This disorder appears to be caused by the inhibition of central dopamine receptors in the hypothalamus, which results in increased heat generation and decreased heat dissipation. The serotonin syndrome, seen with SSRIs, monoamine oxidase inhibitors (MAOIs), and other serotonergic medications, has many overlapping features, including hyperthermia, but may be distinguished by the presence of diarrhoea, tremor, and myoclonus rather than the lead-pipe rigidity of neuroleptic malignant syndrome.

Fauci AS, *et al. Harrison's Principles of Internal Medicine*, 17th edn. McGraw-Hill Medical, 2008.

40. A.   There is a clear link between DSH attempt and suicide, with 15–25% of those who die by suicide having presented with an episode of DSH in the year prior to their death. Between one-third and two-thirds of those who commit suicide having a lifetime history of DSH. About 0.7–1.0% of DSH patients die within a year by suicide. This is approximately 66 times the annual risk of suicide in the general population in the UK. There appears to be marked variability between different groups, with rates of suicide following DSH increasing markedly with age at initial presentation, living alone, and in those with multiple episodes of DSH. Males have almost twice the risk of females of committing suicide following an episode of DSH, especially in the following year.

Lloyd G and Guthrie E. *Handbook of Liaison Psychiatry*, illustrated edition. Cambridge University Press, 2007, p. 247.

41. D.   The American guidelines recommend the use of Clozapine or Quetiapine for the management of psychosis in Parkinson's disease. The guidelines also note that Olanzapine should not be used for the same. With few exceptions, all atypical antipsychotics have comparable efficacy against psychosis and the choice is mainly based on their ease of use and the side-effect profile. Risperidone and olanzapine are associated with sedation. Risperidone can cause considerable worsening of parkinsonism. Olanzapine has been known to worsen cognition and hyperglycaemia in patients with diabetes. A recent Committee on Safety of Medicines warning suggests an increased risk of strokes associated with the use of risperidone and olanzapine in old people. Clozapine has the best evidence for use in Parkinson's as this was the first atypical antipsychotic that came on the market. However, due to the tedious monitoring protocols, it is seldom used in the population, and it has a restricted licence in the UK. Quetiapine is favoured by many psychiatrists because of its better side-effect profile and being as efficacious as Clozapine, at least in one study. Aripiprazole has been shown to worsen Parkinson's disease.

Miyasaki JM, Shannon K, Voon V, *et al.*, Quality Standards Subcommittee of the American Academy of Neurology. Practice parameter: evaluation and treatment of depression, psychosis, and dementia in Parkinson disease an evidence-based review,: report of the Quality Standards Subcommittee of the American Academy of Neurology. Neurology 2006; **667**: 996–1002.
Thanvi BR, Lo TCN and Harsh DP. Psychosis in Parkinson's disease. *Postgraduate Medical Journal* 2005; **81**: 644–646.

42. B.   Sodium valproate is considered a human teratogen. Although several studies have shown rates of neural tube defect of up to 10%, the risk is generally considered between 1% and 2%. The effect of the drug on neural tube development is related to its use 17–30 days post conception, and the risk is dose related. The neural tube defect found in exposed infants is more likely to be lumbosacral rather than anencephalic, which suggests a drug effect on neural crest closure. The risk of Ebstein's anomaly among the offspring of lithium users is 1:1000 (0.1%) to 2:1000 (0.05%), or 20 to 40 times higher than the rate in the general population. The most common toxicity effect in offspring exposed to lithium during labour is the 'floppy baby' syndrome, characterized by cyanosis and hypotonicity. Carbamazepine is also considered a human teratogen. In one prospective study of 35 women treated with carbamazepine during the first trimester, craniofacial defects (11%), fingernail hypoplasia (26%), and developmental delay (20%) were found in live-born offspring. The rate for neural tube defects in that report and others ranged between 0.5% and 1%. Regarding antipsychotics, a recent review showed that both first-generation antipsychotics (FGA) and second-generation antipsychotics (SGA) seem to be associated with an increased risk of neonatal complications. However, most SGAs appear to increase the risk of gestational metabolic complications and babies large for gestational age and with mean birth weight significantly heavier than those exposed to FGAs. These risks have been reported rarely with FGAs. Hence, the choice of the less harmful option in pregnancy should be limited to FGAs in drug-naive patients. When pregnancy occurs during antipsychotic treatment, the choice to continue the previous therapy should be preferred.

Yonkers KA, Wisner KL, Stowe Z, et al. Management of bipolar disorder during pregnancy and the postpartum period. *American Journal of Psychiatry* 2004; **1614**: 608–620.

Morrow J, Russell A, Guthrie, et al. Malformation risks of antiepileptic drugs in pregnancy: a prospective study from the UK Epilepsy and Pregnancy Register. *Journal of Neurology, Neurosurgery, and Psychiatry* 2006; **77**: 193–198.

43. A.   The Center for Disease Control definition of CFS (also called neurasthenia and myalgic encephalitis in the UK) consists of severe unexplained fatigue for over 6 months. This is of new or definite onset; not due to continuing exertion; not resolved by rest; and is functionally impairing. The criterion also mentions other symptoms that are suggestive of CFS, out of which at least four need to be present for the diagnosis. They are impaired memory or concentration; sore throat; tender lymph nodes; muscle pain; pain in several joints; new pattern of headaches; unrefreshing sleep; postexertional malaise lasting more than 24 hours. Although non-refreshing sleep is a criterion, late insomnia is not.

Gelder M, Harrison P, and Cowen P. *Shorter Oxford Textbook of Psychiatry*, 5th edn. Oxford University Press, 2006, p. 387.

44. E.   Two large, multicentre trials were designed to assess the safety, efficacy, and consequence of treating depression in patients with cardiovascular disease. The first, Sertraline Treatment of Major Depression in Patients with Acute MI or Unstable Angina (SADHART) was a randomized, double-blind, placebo-controlled trial conducted in 40 medical centres. The primary objective of SADHART was to evaluate the safety and efficacy of sertraline treatment for major depressive disorder in patients hospitalized for acute MI or unstable angina without other life-threatening medical complications. The results of the study indicated that sertraline was found to be safe and effective in a subgroup of more severely depressed patients. The second multicentre trial, Enhancing Recovery in Coronary Heart Disease Patients (ENRICHD), aimed to determine whether mortality and recurrent infarction are reduced by treatment of depression after an acute MI. Treatment included cognitive behaviour therapy (CBT) and the use of SSRIs when indicated. Similar to the SADHART findings, the interventions did not increase event-free survival; however, they did improve both depression severity and social isolation.

Blumenfield, M and Strain J. *Psychosomatic Medicine*, 1st edn. Lippincott Williams and Wilkins, 2006, p. 56.

45. A.   The term premenstrual syndrome (PMS) was first coined by a physician from England named Katharina Dalton in 1953; however, premenstrual tension was a term used prior to this. More than 150 different symptoms have been attributed to PMS, but the one unifying concept is that these symptoms must occur during the (late) luteal phase of the menstrual cycle, causing significant impairment in a woman's functioning, and must disappear within the first few days of menses. The American Psychiatric Association recognizes premenstrual dysphoric disorder (PMDD) as a subset of PMS that was designed to focus on women with severe symptoms causing marked impairment in functioning. PMDD has a lifetime prevalence of approximately 2–4% in menstruating women. Sixty-five per cent of women with unipolar mood disorder experience PMS, and women with PMS have a 60% lifetime prevalence of major depression. In a recent meta-analysis on the efficacy of SSRIs in PMDD, 15 randomized controlled trials (RCTs) were found demonstrating SSRIs as effective for behavioural and physical symptom amelioration and have the best evidence to date. Other supplements do not have solid research evidence to support their use to date, including vitamin E, vitamin A, magnesium, primrose oil, dong quai, black cohosh, wild yam, St John's wort, or kava.

Wyatt KM, Dimmock PW and O'Brien PMS. Selective serotonin reuptake inhibitors for premenstrual syndrome. Cochrane Database Syst Rev 2004.

Blumenfield M and Strain, J. *Psychosomatic Medicine*, 1st edn. Lippincott Williams & Wilkins, 2006, p. 583.

46. E.   The evidence here is limited and sometimes conflicting. Overall it seems that a current eating disorder, particularly active anorexia nervosa, carries an excess small risk to the mother and the foetus. A recent large cohort study published in the *British Journal of Psychiatry* of women with anorexia nervosa, women with bulimia nervosa, women with both disorders, and controls found that women with bulimia nervosa were significantly more likely to have a history of miscarriage and those with anorexia nervosa were significantly more likely to have smaller babies than the general population. Previous retrospective studies have found that women with a history of an eating disorder had a higher rate of miscarriage, small for gestational age babies, low birth weight babies, babies with microcephaly, intrauterine growth restriction, and premature labour.

Ward VB. Eating disorders in pregnancy. *British Medical Journal*, 2008; **336**: 93–96.

Micali N, Simonoff E and Treasure J. Risk of major adverse perinatal outcomes in women with eating disorders. *British Journal of Psychiatry* 2007; **190**: 255–259.

47. E.   Much of what we know about suicide in the UK psychiatric population is based on data collected by the National Confidential Inquiry into Suicide and Homicide by People with Mental Illness. They are a relatively morbid group – more than half of patients had a secondary psychiatric diagnosis, and 16% of patients had been admitted to a psychiatric bed on more than five occasions. Forty-nine per cent of the patients who died had been in contact with services in the previous week, 19% in the previous 24 hours. At final contact, immediate suicide risk was estimated to be low or absent in 86% of cases. 14% were non-compliant with treatment.

Appleby L, *et al. Avoidable deaths. Five year report of the national confidential inquiry into suicide and homicide by people with mental illness.* The University of Manchester, 2006.

48. B.   Common somatic complaints of pregnancy may be misconstrued as symptoms of depression when using traditional depression assessment scales (such as the Beck Depression Inventory, the Hamilton Rating Scale for Depression, or the Center for Epidemiological Studies Depression Scale), symptoms of depression reported by pregnant women may be misidentified as normal pregnancy-related complaints by treating obstetricians. Use of the 10-item Edinburgh Postnatal Depression Scale has been found to accurately identify depression in pregnant and postpartum women. This brief screening instrument has been validated in pregnant and postpartum populations and is easily incorporated for standard practice use in obstetrical treatment settings.

Kaplan HI. *Kaplan and Sadock's Comprehensive Textbook of Psychiatry*, 8th edn. Lippincott Williams & Wilkins, 2004 p. 2306.

49. E.   Suicide rates are increased in all psychiatric disorders, except dementia. Most estimates of the lifetime suicide rate in schizophrenia are in the region of 5% to 10%, slightly less than in major affective disorders. The long-term risk of suicide in primary affective disorder has been estimated at 15%. Suicidal behaviour is most common among patients with depression, alcoholism or substance abuse, schizophrenia, and personality disorder. Anxiety disorders were found to be independently associated with a more than doubled risk of past and future suicidal ideation and behaviour.

Lloyd G and Guthrie E. *Handbook of Liaison Psychiatry*, illustrated edition. Cambridge University Press, 2007, p. 249.

Sareen J, Cox BJ, Afifi TO, *et al.* Anxiety disorders and risk for suicidal ideation and suicide attempts: a population-based longitudinal study of adults. *Archives of General Psychiatry* 2005; **62**: 1249–1257.

50. C.   The most common constellation of mood symptoms experienced by women in the immediate postpartum period is typically referred to as the postpartum blues or baby blues. A relatively common phenomenon (occurring in 50–80% of women), postpartum blues include transient symptoms and rapid mood shifts, including tearfulness, irritability, anxiety, insomnia, lack of energy, loss of appetite, and the general experience of feeling overwhelmed particularly with regard to newborn care-giving tasks. By definition, the postpartum blues are transient in nature. Onset typically occurs after the third postpartum day, after the mother has left the hospital after delivery. Symptoms typically peak by day 5 and spontaneously resolve by day 10 postpartum. It has been estimated that 75% of women who experience symptoms of postpartum blues will display such a time-limited course; however, 20–25% may go on to experience full-blown postpartum depression.

Kaplan HI. *Kaplan and Sadock's Comprehensive Textbook of Psychiatry*, 8th edn. Lippincott Williams & Wilkins, 2004 p. 2308.

1. **Lisa is a 35-year-old lady, diagnosed with depression. She has been referred by her psychiatrist for psychodynamic psychotherapy. According to her therapist, Lisa has the ability to conceive of her own mental state as explanations of her behaviour. This phenomenon is called**
   A. Transference
   B. Mentalization
   C. Counter transference
   D. Empathy
   E. None of the above

2. **Which of the following suggests sufficient psychological mindedness in Lisa?**
   A. She needs a lot of prompts to give her story
   B. She finds it difficult to bring up memories with appropriate affect
   C. She is unaware of this unconscious mental life
   D. She does not have poor self-esteem
   E. She is unable to step back and observe reflectively

3. **During her first session, Lisa asks her therapist about certain terms she came across on the internet. "What is transference?"**
   A. Empathy in relationships
   B. Therapist's response to the patient based on the therapist's previous relationships
   C. Patient's response to the therapist based on the patient's previous relationships
   D. Transfer of positive thoughts from the therapist to the patient through self-disclosure
   E. All of the above

4. **Which of the following correctly describes counter-transference?**
   A. The analyst's or psychotherapist's transference reactions to the patient
   B. His or her reactions to the patient's transferences
   C. Any reactions, feelings and attitudes of the analyst or therapist towards the patient, regardless of their source.
   D. All of the above
   E. None of the above

5. During the psychotherapy sessions, the therapist notes that Lisa uses a number of defence mechanisms that are classified as 'mature defences' according to Vaillant. Which of the following is a mature defence?

   A. Suppression
   B. Repression
   C. Dissociation
   D. Passive aggression
   E. Denial

6. Nearing the end of her therapy session, Lisa blurts out 'I am abusing my children' before quickly shifting the topic to other things. What is the most immediate appropriate thing for the therapist to do?

   A. End the session on time and explore it in the next session
   B. Ask her what she meant by 'abusing'
   C. Reassure her that everything said in therapy is confidential
   D. Tell her that you have to report her to the social services
   E. Carry out an extensive assessment of risk to the child

7. Which of the following represents the concept of borderline personality organization?

   A. Identity diffusion
   B. Utilizing primitive defences
   C. Intact reality testing
   D. Characteristic splitting in object relations
   E. All of the above

8. In dynamic psychotherapy, the therapist at times uses certain techniques that represent the 'supportive' end of the psychodynamic continuum rather than the 'expressive' end. Which of the following is suggestive of a 'supportive' technique?

   A. Confrontation
   B. Clarification
   C. Interpretation
   D. Interpretation of transference
   E. Giving advice

9. The process by which unconscious ideas are repressed and prevented from reaching awareness because they are unacceptable in psychotherapy is called

   A. Transference
   B. Counter-transference
   C. Resistance
   D. Therapeutic alliance
   E. Repression

10. Jack is a 35-year-old man who perceived his parents as overly authoritarian. His therapist on the other hand, is friendly and non-authoritarian, but at times firm and sets definite limits. The attitude of his therapist gave Jack the opportunity to identify with a new parent figure. This is an example of a process described by Franz Alexander. Which of the following terms best represents this process?

    A. Resistance
    B. Counter-transference
    C. Corrective emotional experience
    D. Therapeutic alliance
    E. Childhood neurosis

11. Nick has been diagnosed with major depression. His GP is considering referring Nick for psychodynamic psychotherapy. According to the GP, Nick has certain qualities he thinks are important for a good prognosis in psychodynamic psychotherapy. Which of the qualities shown by Nick has been shown NOT to predict good response in psychodynamic psychotherapy?

    A. Psychological mindedness
    B. Introspectiveness
    C. Acting out affects
    D. Reasonable object relationships
    E. Intense search for understanding

12. Brief psychodynamic psychotherapy has been shown NOT to be of benefit in which of the following conditions?

    A. Panic disorder
    B. Severe depression
    C. Interpersonal difficulties
    D. Opiate dependence
    E. Somatoform disorder

13. Which of the following therapies involve 'strokes' that people exchange and 'games' that people play?

    A. Person-centred psychotherapy
    B. Gestalt therapy
    C. Transactional analysis
    D. Existential therapy
    E. Physiotherapy

14. Focusing on a detail out of context while ignoring other, more salient features in the situation is called

    A. Arbitrary interference
    B. Selective abstraction
    C. Overgeneralization
    D. Dichotomous thinking
    E. Personalization

15. **Global, rigid, absolute, and overgeneralized convictions about the self that have powerful effects on how we perceive ourselves are called**

A. Core beliefs
B. Conditional rules
C. Automatic thoughts
D. Intermediate beliefs
E. None of the above

16. **Which of the following terms refer to beliefs that thoughts and behaviours have reciprocal and equivalent effects?**

A. Anxiety sensitivity
B. Pathological worry
C. Thought–action fusion (TAF)
D. Intolerance of uncertainty
E. None of the above

17. **Which of the following is a technique for automatic thought modification?**

A. Guided discovery
B. Recognizing mood shifts
C. Checklists for automatic thoughts
D. Imagery
E. Examining the evidence

18. **A woman comes to your outpatient clinic. She has recurrent thoughts of contamination with germs and has to wash her hands up to 20 times every time she touches wooden surfaces. This prevents her from looking after her 2-year-old child. She is worried that the child may not be gaining the required weight. She has also started to lose the skin of her palms due to the excessive washing. The treatment you would recommend would be**

A. Cognitive behaviour therapy (CBT)
B. Combination of selective serotonin reuptake inhibitors (SSRIs) and CBT
C. SSRI only
D. Psychodynamic therapy
E. Eye movement desensitization therapy (EMDR)

19. **Jack has certain core beliefs about being unlovable. He thinks that this characteristic makes people abandon him. In order to avoid this, he turns out to be excessively self-sacrificing to his family. From a schema-based therapy point of view, what is the underlying cognitive process that is maintaining the schema?**

A. Schema surrender
B. Schema compensation
C. Schema avoidance
D. Schema utilization
E. None of the above

20. **Maria has obsessive thoughts of a violent nature towards her mother. Which of the following is the least characteristic of dysfunctional assumptions likely to be seen in Maria?**

   A. Having a thought about stabbing my mother is like doing it
   B. I should exercise control over my thoughts
   C. Although I believe that I will not hurt my mother, I am still responsible for this harmful thought
   D. Not neutralizing the thought of stabbing her mother is equivalent to wishing her mother stabbed
   E. If I don't please everyone, I am a failure

21. **Covert sensitisation is best used in the treatment of which of the following**

   A. Alcohol dependence
   B. Panic disorder
   C. Generalized anxiety disorder
   D. OCD
   E. Major depressive disorder

22. **Parent management training is based on the principles of**

   A. Psychoanalysis
   B. Learning theory
   C. Systems theory of family therapy
   D. Object relations theory
   E. Play therapy

23. **Which of the following is the first step in systematic desensitization?**

   A. Constructing a hierarchy
   B. Relaxation training
   C. Exposure *in vivo*
   D. Exposure *in vitro*
   E. Flooding

24. **Habit reversal components include all the following except**

   A. Training to be aware of onset
   B. Training in thought stopping
   C. Training in initiating competing response
   D. Relaxation
   E. Social support

25. **Orgasmic reconditioning is used in**

   A. Premature ejaculation
   B. Erectile dysfunction
   C. Delayed ejaculation
   D. Changing sexual preferences
   E. None of the above

26. Massed negative practice treatment is used in the treatment of

A. Tic disorder
B. OCD
C. Generalized anxiety disorder
D. Panic disorder
E. None of the above

27. Token economy programmes are based on which of the following psychological principle?

A. Classical conditioning
B. Operant conditioning
C. Vicarious learning
D. Aversive conditioning
E. None of the above

28. Dawn is known to have moderate learning disability. She hits her head very often with her right hand. Her therapist teaches Dawn to engage in knitting with her right hand. This gradually replaced her maladaptive behaviour. The process through which the therapist replaced a maladaptive behaviour with an adaptive constructive one is through the principles of

A. Positive behavioural programming
B. Massed negative practice treatment
C. Functional communications training
D. Habit reversal programme
E. None of the above

29. Which of the following in the least likely outcome in a patient undergoing CBT for hypochondriasis?

A. Decrease in hypochondriacal thoughts
B. Better social role functioning
C. Less distress at thoughts of illness
D. Decrease in health-related anxiety
E. Remission of hypochondriacal somatic symptoms

30. Which of the following approaches have shown to be the most effective in bulimia nervosa?

A. CBT
B. Interpersonal psychotherapy (IPT)
C. Psychodynamic psychotherapy
D. Family therapy
E. Exposure and response prevention.

31. **How would you treat an intelligent 15-year-old boy with moderate depression but no suicidal thoughts?**

    A. CBT
    B. SSRI and CBT
    C. TCA alone
    D. TCA and CBT
    E. SSRI alone

32. **The therapeutic work of interpersonal psychotherapy is organized around central interpersonal problem areas in the patient's life. Which of the following situations are possible problem areas in a case of acute depression?**

    A. Role transition
    B. Grief
    C. Role dispute
    D. Interpersonal deficits
    E. All of the above

33. **Which of the following is NOT a step in interpersonal psychotherapy for depression?**

    A. Evaluating depressed mood
    B. Evaluating interpersonal relationships
    C. Employing thought records
    D. Improving capacity to communicate
    E. Enhancing understanding of depression as a medical illness

34. **In the landmark National Institute of Mental Health (NIMH) Treatment of Depression Collaborative Research Program, which of the following psychotherapies was found to be equivalent to imipramine in severe depression?**

    A. CBT
    B. IPT
    C. Psychodynamic psychotherapy
    D. Family therapy
    E. All of the above

35. **Which of the following is the first step involved in crisis intervention?**

    A. Patient is encouraged to consider solutions
    B. Assess the patient's problems and assets
    C. Test the solutions
    D. Reduce arousal
    E. Consider future coping mechanisms

36. **Dialectical behavioural therapy uses all of the following techniques except**

    A. Cognitive behavioural techniques
    B. Mindfulness techniques
    C. Aphorisms
    D. Role reversal
    E. Dialectical techniques

37. **Which of the following is considered to be the most important therapeutic factor in group psychotherapy?**

    A. Ventilation of affect
    B. Pairing
    C. Cohesion
    D. Dependence
    E. Discussion

38. **In a therapeutic community, the members tolerate behaviour that may not be accepted anywhere else. This process is called**

    A. Permissiveness
    B. Cohesion
    C. Mutual help
    D. Imitation
    E. Altruism

39. **In a family therapy session, the mother is asked to comment on the relationship between her husband and their eldest son. After this, the family members are asked to comment on the mother's response. This method is called**

    A. Paradoxical injunction
    B. Circular questioning
    C. Socratic questioning
    D. Role reversal
    E. Sculpting

40. **Which of the following is not a goal of family therapy?**

    A. Improving communication
    B. Improving agreement on roles of each member
    C. Improving cognitive style
    D. Decreasing conflict among members
    E. Decreasing distress in the member considered to be the patient

41. **Traps, dilemmas, and snags are techniques typically used in**

    A. Cognitive analytical therapy
    B. Cognitive behavioural therapy
    C. Rational emotive therapy
    D. Interpersonal therapy
    E. Psychodynamic psychotherapy

42. **Which of the following statements accurately describes collaborative empiricism in CBT?**
    A. A relationship in which the client is presumed to be right in his or her assumptions and the therapist collaborates to reduce the impact of the assumptions
    B. A relationship in which the therapy is considered empirical with no guaranteed positive outcome in order to avoid later disappointment
    C. A relationship in which the therapist and client share their problems with each other and collaborate to find mutual solutions
    D. A relationship in which the therapist and the client work as partners in identifying and modifying dysfunctional cognitions and behaviours.
    E. A relationship in which the client agrees for the therapist to share information with multiple other therapists who offer different models of therapy

43. **A method of group psychotherapy where members of the group take on the roles of 'the protagonist' and 'auxillary ego' while the therapist takes on the role of 'the director' is**
    A. Drama therapy
    B. Biofeedback therapy
    C. Psychodrama
    D. Direction group
    E. Auxillary ego therapy

44. **Justin is a medical student who faints every time he encounters medical situations involving blood or injury. His therapist trains him to tense the muscles of the arms, legs, and torso at the earliest signs of faintness. This type of therapy is called**
    A. Applied relaxation
    B. Applied tension
    C. Autogenic training
    D. Biofeedback
    E. Self-hypnosis

45. **The acronym 'FRAMES' in brief intervention for alcohol dependence stands for all except**
    A. Feedback
    B. Roll with resistance
    C. Advice
    D. Empathic interviewing
    E. Self-efficacy

46. **In the treatment of borderline personality disorder, which of the following does Stage 2 of dialectical behaviour therapy target?**
    A. Severe behavioural dyscontrol
    B. Quiet desperation
    C. Problematic patterns in living
    D. Incompleteness
    E. None of the above

47. Rachel is a 35-year-old woman who was recently involved in a life-threatening road traffic accident. She developed symptoms suggestive of post-traumatic stress disorder (PTSD) over a period of a month following the accident. The symptoms interfered with her daily activities. She refused to drive to work and started missing her work. She also stopped taking her children to the nursery. According to NICE guidelines, what treatment is recommended?

   A. Trauma-focused CBT
   B. Single-session debriefing
   C. Wait and watch
   D. EMDR
   E. Relaxation therapy

48. During a biofeedback session, which of the following denotes a stage of relaxation?

   A. Increase in beta waves on EEG
   B. Decrease in skin conductance
   C. Decrease in skin temperature
   D. Increase in action potential recordings on the electromyogram (EMG)
   E. All of the above

49. Cognitive therapy aims to modify the schemas that perpetuate depression or anxiety. Which of the following is least likely with respect to schemas?

   A. Schemas contain basic rules for screening, filtering, and processing external information
   B. Schemas are behaviours representative of the patient's presenting problem
   C. Conditional rules such as 'if–then' statements can serve as dysfunctional schemas
   D. Schemas include core beliefs about oneself
   E. Simple schemas can exist without influencing psychopathology

50. On the basis of cognitive theory, certain cognitive distortions are formulated to explain both behavioural features and bodily symptoms of various psychiatric disorders. Which of the following themes is correctly matched with the disorder?

   A. Hopelessness: panic disorder
   B. Sense of failure: agoraphobia
   C. Attentional bias towards threat: generalized anxiety disorder
   D. Black and white thinking: schizophrenia
   E. Minimization of positive appraisal: specific phobias

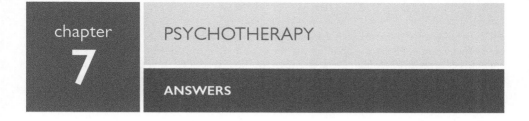

1. B. The capacity for mentalizing grows out of attachment theory and refers to a person's ability to conceive of his or her own and others' mental states as explanations of behaviour. Hence, it is related to psychological mindedness. The psychodynamic clinician assesses the ability of a patient to see that his or her behaviour grows out of a set of beliefs, feelings, and perspectives that are not necessarily the same as others'. Like empathy, mentalizing requires a capacity to sense what is going on in another's mind and respond accordingly. This capacity to be sensitive to what others are feeling and to know that one's internal states contribute to one's behaviour augurs well for a more exploratory or interpretative approach in dynamic psychotherapy.

Gabbard GO. *Textbook of Psychotherapeutic Treatments in Psychiatry*, 1st edn. American Psychiatric Publishing, 2008, p 29.

2. D. According to Nina Coltart, during psychotherapy, a therapist is exercising his/her skills and psychological mindedness to explore the patient's psyche. If the patient is also psychologically minded, the prospects of treatment success are thought to be greatly increased. Whether a patient is psychologically minded depends on a number of characters. They include:

1. The capacity to give a history that deepens, acquires more coherence, and becomes texturally more substantial as it goes on.
2. The capacity to give such a history without needing too much prompting, and a history which gives the listener an increasing awareness that the patient feels currently related in him/herself, to his/her own story.
3. The capacity to bring up memories with appropriate affects.
4. Some awareness in the patient that he has an unconscious mental life.
5. Some capacity to step back, if only momentarily, from self-experience, and to observe it reflectively.
6. The capacity, or more strongly a wish, to accept and handle increased responsibility for the self.
7. The capacity to imagine and dream and use metaphors.
8. Some capacity for achievement, and some realistic self-esteem.

Coltart N. The assessment of psychological-mindedness in the diagnostic interview. *British Journal of Psychiatry* 1988; **153**: 819–820.

Naismith J and Grant S. *Seminars in the Psychotherapies*. Gaskell, 2007, p. 8.

3. C. Transference is the displacement of feelings and thoughts associated with a figure in the patient's past onto the therapist. Transference is often unconscious, at least initially, and the patient is often puzzled by their behaviour towards the therapist because it does not make sense, based on who the therapist really is. Hence the enactment of missing a session or of coming late to a session may reveal unconscious transference. The prevailing view about transference is that the therapist's actual behaviour always influences the patient's experience of the therapist. Hence the transference to the therapist is partly based on real characteristics and partly on figures from the patient's past: a combination of old and new relationships. Many therapists believe that interpretation of this transference is an essential process of psychodynamic psychotherapy. Gabbard says that one should postpone the interpretation of transference until it becomes a resistance and until it is close to the patient's awareness. In other words, if things are going reasonably well, it makes no sense to interpret transference. If the patient develops, for example, erotized or highly negative feelings, which impede the process of the therapy, interpretation may be essential. Many therapists regard treatment that focuses on transference as more exploratory than therapy geared to extra-transference relationships. In supportive therapy, interpretation of the transference may be minimized, although the therapist may silently interpret the transference as a way of increasing his or her understanding of the patient.

Gabbard GO. *Textbook of Psychotherapeutic Treatments in Psychiatry*, 1st edn. American Psychiatric Publishing, 2008, p. 56.

Tasman A, Maj M, First M B, *et al. Psychiatry*, 3rd edn. WileyBlackwell, 2008, p. 1854.

4. D. Freud used the term counter-transference to describe the analyst's transference towards the patient. In other words, the patient might remind the therapist of someone from the therapist's past, so that the therapist starts to treat the patient as though he or she were that figure. Over time, this view of counter-transference was broadened to include the total emotional reaction of the therapist to the patient. Today it is recognized that counter-transference is jointly created—it partly involves the therapist's past relationships, but it also involves feelings induced in the therapist by the patient's behaviour. Counter-transference is variously defined as (1) the analyst's or psychotherapist's transference reactions to the patient; (2) his or her reactions to the patient's transferences; and (3) any reactions, feelings and attitudes of the analyst or therapist toward the patient, regardless of their source. These responses are manifestations of the requisite engagement by the therapist or analyst in the emotional process of treatment. Moreover, these reactions are a rich source of understanding of the patient's experience as it touches the therapist affectively.

Gabbard GO. *Textbook of Psychotherapeutic Treatments in Psychiatry*, 1st edn. American Psychiatric Publishing, 2008, p. 58.

Tasman A, Maj M, First MB, *et al. Psychiatry*, 3rd edn. WileyBlackwell, 2008, p. 1854.

5. A. George Vaillant classified defences hierarchically according to the relative degree of maturity associated with them. Narcissistic defences (denial, distortion, and projection) are the most primitive and appear in children and persons who are psychotically disturbed. Immature defences (acting out, passive-aggression, blocking, introjection, and regression) are seen in adolescents and some non-psychotic patients. Neurotic defences (dissociation, displacement, intellectualization, isolation, reaction formation, and repression) are encountered in obsessive–compulsive and hysterical patients as well as in adults under stress. Mature defences according to Vaillant are altruism, anticipation, asceticism, humour, sublimation, and suppression. These mechanisms often are used in healthy coping mechanisms.

Sadock BJ and Sadock VA. (). *Kaplan and Sadock's Synopsis of Psychiatry: Behavioral Sciences/clinical Psychiatry*, 10th edn. Lippincott Williams & Wilkins, 2007, p. 206.

6. B. In the USA, therapists have a legal duty to warn and protect third parties endangered by their patients. In the UK, there is no binding requirement on clinicians to disclose dangerousness. The decision to disclose is based on the judgement that the responsibility to protect the public outweighs the duty to the patient to protect confidentiality. The clinician has the responsibility to make a considered decision whether or not to infringe the right to confidentiality. Statute law (e.g. notification of diseases) determines when the clinician 'must' infringe that right; case law when he 'may' do so. Most psychotherapy falls under the latter. Each case must be considered on its merits, possibly on the basis of a risk assessment, and where there is a doubt, the clinician must discuss it with another clinician. In any case, welfare of children is of foremost importance. In this particular case, Lisa said she was abusing her children. We do not know what she meant by 'abuse'. So, as common sense would inform, the first step is for the therapist to confirm what she means by 'abuse'. If there is a need, the next step would be an informed risk assessment. Confidentiality and disclosure are usually discussed with the patient before therapy. Since there is a potential risk to children, ending the session and reassuring Lisa about confidentiality are obviously wrong choices. Premature reporting to social services would result in unnecessary labelling and also possible loss of rapport and therapeutic alliance. Criticizing her would also lead to a break in the therapeutic relationship and would be against the principles of 'unconditional positive regard'. If there is a case for disclosure, the patient herself should be encouraged to disclose to social services, as this would be in the best interests of the children involved and the patient. It is generally thought that inexperienced staff and students should not enquire about abuse or ask known victims about details of their experience, although they may be approached by patients making tentative attempts at disclosure, the general rule must be that inexperienced individuals should not invite discussion of a sensitive subject such as sexual abuse unless they are being supervised and trained to deal with it. In this case, it is thought that the psychotherapist is being supervised and would do a general risk assessment based on history and mental state.

Gabbard GO, Beck JS, and Holmes J. *Oxford Textbook of Psychotherapy*. Oxford University Press, 2007, p. 488.

Babiker IE. Managing sexual abuse disclosure by adult psychiatric patients – some suggestions. *Psychiatric Bulletin* 1993; **17**: 286–288.

7. E.   Otto Kernberg proposed the term 'borderline personality organization' (BPO), a broad concept encompassing all severe personality disorders. BPO is a stable permanent state based on four criteria: diffuse identity; primitive defences, including splitting, projection, and projective identification; intact reality testing that is prone to alterations and failures because of aggression; and object relations characterized by splitting. The term 'Identity diffusion' was developed by Erikson and later used by Kernberg in his concept of BPO. In psychodynamic terms an individual with identity diffusion has not integrated good self-images with bad, and, instead, has multiple, contradictory self-images, some good, some bad. These are invoked at different times and in different situations so that a meaningful, integrated image of the self is never formed. Salman Akhtar delineates the syndrome of identity diffusion as consisting of six clinical features: (1) contradictory character traits, (2) temporal discontinuity in the self, (3) lack of authenticity, (4) feelings of emptiness, (5) gender dysphoria, and (6) inordinate ethnic and moral relativism. This syndrome implies severe personality pathology. The inner world in BPO according to Kernberg, is characterized by split objects. Instead of stable and smoothly integrated internal representations of people and their relationships, the self and others are experienced in contrasts of either black or white – 'no grey zones'. These people generally have an intact reality testing, but are prone to breaks in it, leading to the so-called 'micropsychotic' episodes.

S Akhtar. The syndrome of identity diffusion. *American Journal of Psychiatry* 1984; **141**: 1381–1385.

Gabbard GO, Beck JS, and Holmes J (). *Oxford Textbook of Psychotherapy*. Oxford University Press 2007, p. 292.

Bruce-Jones W and Coid J. Identity diffusion presenting as multiple personality disorder in a female psychopath. *British Journal of Psychiatry* 1992; **160**: 541–544.

8. E.   Dynamic (psychoanalytic) psychotherapy is often conceptualised as being on a continuum of expressive to supportive. Traditionally, psychoanalytic psychotherapy has focused on the recovery of repressed psychological material. This process has been called 'expressive' and is distinguished from the 'supportive' psychotherapies, which concentrate on supporting healthy defence (coping) mechanisms. The therapist may employ more or less expressive and supportive interventions, depending on the needs of the patient. Among the given responses in the question, advice giving leans towards the supportive end of the continuum. In addition to advice giving, other techniques usually employed that are at the supportive end of the continuum are praise, suggestions, reassurance, environmental intervention, and manipulation.

Sadock BJ and Sadock VA. Kaplan and Sadock's Synopsis of Psychiatry: Behavioral Sciences/clinical Psychiatry, 10th edn. Lippincott Williams & Wilkins, 2007, p. 928.

Tasman A, Maj M, First MB, et al. (). *Psychiatry*, 3rd edn. WileyBlackwell, 2008, p. 1852.

9. C.   Resistance is broadly defined as the conscious or, more often, unconscious force within the patient opposing the emergence of unconscious material. Resistance is thought of as the patient's attempt to protect her or himself by avoiding the anticipated emotional discomfort that accompanies the emergence of conflictual, dangerous, or painful experiences, feelings, thoughts, memories, needs, and desires. Resistance occurs through the use of unconscious defence mechanisms. The recognition, clarification, and interpretation of resistance constitute important activities of the psychoanalyst and the psychoanalytic psychotherapist, both of whom must first appreciate how a patient is warding off anxiety before understanding why he or she is so compelled.

Sadock BJ and Sadock VA. Kaplan and Sadock's Synopsis of Psychiatry: Behavioral Sciences/clinical Psychiatry, 10th edn. Lippincott Williams & Wilkins, 2007, p. 926.

10. C. The therapeutic relationship between therapist and patient gives a therapist an opportunity to display behaviour different from the destructive or unproductive behaviour of a patient's parent. At times, such experiences seem to neutralize or reverse some effects of the parents' mistakes. If the patient had overly authoritarian parents, the therapist's friendly, flexible, non-judgemental, non-authoritarian, but at times firm and limit-setting attitude gives the patient an opportunity to adjust to, be led by, and identify with a new parent figure. Franz Alexander described this process as a corrective emotional experience. It draws on elements of both psychoanalysis and psychoanalytic psychotherapy.

Sadock BJ and Sadock VA. *Kaplan and Sadock's Synopsis of Psychiatry: Behavioral Sciences/clinical Psychiatry*, 10th edn. Lippincott Williams & Wilkins, 2007, p. 931.

11. C. Most psychotherapists consider certain qualities in their patients as prerequisites for engaging in psychodynamic psychotherapy. These include psychological mindedness: curiosity about oneself and the capacity for self-scrutiny. Those who are unable to articulate and comprehend their inner thoughts and feelings cannot negotiate with the fundamental analytical words and their meanings. The inability to examine one's own motivations and behaviours precludes benefits from the analytical method. Introspectiveness: the person should be able to experience and learn from intense affects or conflicts without acting them out. The person should be able to form reasonable object relationships, usually the capacity to form and maintain, as well as to detach from, a trusting object relationship is essential. High motivation: the patient needs a strong motivation to persevere, in light of the rigors of intense and lengthy treatment. The desire for health and self-understanding must surpass the neurotic need for unhappiness. The person should be able to tolerate frustration and therapeutic regression.

Sadock BJ and Sadock VA. Kaplan and Sadock's Synopsis of Psychiatry: Behavioral Sciences/clinical Psychiatry, 10th edn. Lippincott Williams & Wilkins, 2007, p. 926.
Tasman A, Maj M, First MB, *et al. Psychiatry*, 3rd edn. WileyBlackwell, 2008, p. 1862.

12. B. Inclusion criteria for brief psychodynamic psychotherapy diagnoses: depression, mild to moderate; anxiety, post-traumatic stress disorder, social, panic; somatoform disorders; eating disorders; opiate dependence;. Patient characteristics include good object relationships (has had at least one relationship); highly motivated, 'willing' patient; narrow symptom/problem focus; interpersonal difficulties. Exclusion criteria for brief psychodynamic psychotherapy include a diagnosis of severe depression, bipolar disorder, psychosis, suicidality; obsessive compulsive disorder (OCD); severe somatizing disorders; severe eating disorders; poor object relationships; poor motivation; chronic, severe character pathology; diffuse, ill-defined symptomatology. Most of the above criteria are derived from a systematic review of psychodynamic psychotherapies by Leichsenring in 2005.

Gabbard GO. *Textbook of Psychotherapeutic Treatments in Psychiatry*, 1st edn. American Psychiatric Publishing, 2008, p. 73.
Leichsenring F. (2005). Are psychodynamic and psychoanalytic therapies effective? A review of empirical data. *International Journal of Psycho-Analysis* **86**: 841–868.

13. C.   Transactional analysis developed by Eric Berne in 1960s. According to Berne, transactions are stimuli presented by one person that evoke a corresponding response in another. Berne defined psychological 'games' as stereotyped and predictable transactions that people learn in childhood and continue to play throughout their lives. Strokes, the basic motivating factors of human behaviour consist of specific rewards such as approval and love. All people have three ego states that exist within them: the child (the primitive element), the adult (the reality element), and the parent (an introject of the values of a person's actual parents). The therapeutic process helps people to understand whether they are functioning in a child, adult or parent mode when interacting with others. It is thought that as patients learn to recognize characteristic games being repeated throughout life, they can ultimately function in the adult mode as much as possible in interpersonal relationships.

Sadock BJ and Sadock VA. Kaplan and Sadock's Synopsis of Psychiatry: Behavioral Sciences/clinical Psychiatry, 10th edn. Lippincott Williams & Wilkins, 2007, p. 216.

Freeman C and Power M (). Handbook of Evidence-based Psychotherapies: A Guide for Research and Practice, 1st edn. WileyBlackwell 2007, p. 129.

14. B.   The statement refers to selective abstraction, one of the cognitive biases seen in depression. Other cognitive biases include arbitrary inference, drawing a specific conclusion in the absence of evidence or when the evidence is contrary to the conclusion; overgeneralization, drawing a conclusion on the basis of one or more isolated incidents; dichotomous thinking, the tendency to classify experience in one of two extreme categories, ignoring more moderate variations; personalization, the tendency to relate external events to oneself; magnification/minimization,- exaggerating (i.e. catastrophizing) or belittling the significance or magnitude of an event.

Gabbard GO. Textbook of Psychotherapeutic Treatments in Psychiatry, 1st edn. American Psychiatric Publishing, 2008, p. 173.

15. A.   Core beliefs are global, rigid, absolute, and overgeneralized convictions about the self, others, and the personal world that have powerful effects on how we perceive ourselves and our context. They often have their root in early childhood development. An example of core beliefs is 'I'm incompetent'. These lie dormant until they are activated by certain situations (which reflect childhood events that laid down the core belief). At the next level are 'intermediate thoughts', which consist of rules, assumptions, and attitudes that we use to evaluate ourselves as well as other people and personal experiences. On most occasions, these rules tend to contradict the core belief (in a way reinforcing them). Examples of intermediary beliefs might be 'I need to succeed in everything I do, in order for me to be seen as competent'. A special class of intermediary beliefs is the conditional rule, which takes the form of 'If … then' statements (e.g. 'If I succeed in everything I do, only then others will consider me competent'). Automatic thoughts are cognitions that intervene between external events and a person's emotional reaction to the event. For example, the belief that people will laugh at me when I don't get a distinction at the exam is an automatic thought that occurs to someone who has the aforementioned 'core belief'.

Gabbard GO. Textbook of Psychotherapeutic Treatments in Psychiatry, 1st edn. American Psychiatric Publishing, 2008, p. 171.

16. C. TAF is a cognitive distortion. It is thought to have two forms: 'probability TAF' in which the intrusive thought is believed to increase the probability that a specific negative event will occur. This is prominent in those with violent obsessions. 'Morality TAF' in which experiencing the intrusive thoughts is morally equivalent to carrying out a prohibited action. This distortion is especially prominent in obsessions, is closely related to guilt, and is associated with subsequent attempts at neutralization. A comparable cognitive distortion termed 'thought–shape fusion' is thought to be present in a minority of people with eating problems and occurs when the thought of eating induces feelings of fatness, moral unacceptability, and weight gain. These cognitive distortions can be manipulated experimentally and have clinical implications that include improvement in understanding the nature of the disorder and its treatment.

Rachman S and Shafran R. Cognitive distortions: thought-action fusion. *Clinical Psychology and Psychotherapy* 1999; **6**: 80–85.

17. E. Examining the evidence is a technique in which the therapist and patient collaboratively explore the evidence for and the evidence against a specific distorted thought or belief. When working through the exercise, the therapist asks the patient to write the thought or belief at the top of a piece of paper and then label two columns with 'evidence for' and 'evidence against' the thought. The patient is then guided to explore methodically and write down each piece of evidence. At the end of this procedure, the evidence for and against the cognition is quantified and estimated. Guided discovery is the most frequently used technique to help patients articulate automatic thoughts in sessions. The specific technique used is called Socratic questioning. One of the most powerful ways of teaching patients to detect automatic thoughts is to find a real-life example of how automatic thoughts influence their emotional responses. A shift in mood during the therapy session can be an opportune time for the therapist to facilitate the identification of automatic thoughts. The Automatic Thoughts Questionnaire devised by Hollon and Kendall is a comprehensive list of dysfunctional thoughts that has been used primarily in research studies. Similar lists can be used in clinical settings when patients are having difficulty detecting their automatic thoughts. Imagery and role-play are two methods for uncovering cognitions when direct questions are unsuccessful (or partially successful) in generating suspected automatic thinking.

Gabbard GO. *Textbook of Psychotherapeutic Treatments in Psychiatry*, 1st edn. American Psychiatric Publishing, 2008, p. 208.
Hollon SD and Kendall PC (1980) Cognitive self-statements in depression: development of an automatic thoughts questionnaire. *Cognitive Therapy and Research* **4**: 383–395.

18. B. According to NICE guidelines, in the initial treatment of adults with OCD, low-intensity psychological treatments (including exposure and response prevention (ERP)) (up to 10 therapist hours per patient) should be offered if the patient's degree of functional impairment is mild and/or the patient expresses a preference for a low-intensity approach. These include brief individual CBT (including ERP) using structured self-help materials; brief individual CBT (including ERP) by telephone; group CBT (including ERP) (note, the patient may receive more than 10 hours of therapy in this format). Those with mild functional impairment who are unable to engage in low intensity CBT (including ERP), or for whom low-intensity treatment has proved to be inadequate, should be offered the choice of either a course of an SSRI or more intensive CBT (including ERP) (more than 10 therapist hours per patient). Adults with OCD with moderate functional impairment should be offered the choice of either a course of an SSRI or more intensive CBT (including ERP) (more than 10 therapist hours per patient). Adults with OCD with severe functional impairment should be offered combined treatment with an SSRI and CBT (including ERP).

NICE. CG31 Obsessive-compulsive disorder: NICE guideline. Clinical Guidelines (accessed 7 June 7 2009 http://guidance.nice.org.uk/CG31/NiceGuidance/pdf/English).

19. B. Schema-based approaches in cognitive therapy are based on the original ideas of Beck. Early life experiences produce a number of thought patterns or schemata. These thought patterns are like 'block moulds' into which thoughts fit in when evaluating events. They are otherwise called core beliefs. These result in underlying 'assumptions' which reinforce the core beliefs and from these arise the negative automatic thoughts. Schemata are thought to be dormant, and get activated during a depressive episode. Schemata are patterns of unconditional beliefs that are hard to access and are self-maintaining. There are thought to be three main processes that maintain schemata. Schema surrender is the process where the person seeks evidence that supports the beliefs and dismisses any evidence to the contrary. Schema compensation refers to compensating for the core belief by doing the exact opposite, but, ultimately, this action acts as a reinforcer that maintains the schema, as in the case described in the question. Ultimately, the person believes that the family loves him only because he is self-sacrificing, and if he was not, he would still remain unlovable. Schema avoidance is a group of blocking behaviours that help avoid emotional arousal – e.g. comfort eating.

Naismith J and Grant S. *Seminars in the Psychotherapies.* Gaskell, 2007, p. 149.

20. E. Salkovskis described five characteristic dysfunctional assumptions in patients with obsessive compulsive disorder (OCD). The first option refers to thought–action fusion, i.e. having a thought equates to performing the action. This is consistent with the thoughts of patients with OCD, especially those who have 'violent' obsessions. The second statement that a person should (and can) exercise control over one's thoughts is also consistent with thoughts in OCD. Responsibility is not attenuated by other factors (e.g. the low probability of occurrence) is a typical assumption in patients with OCD. The fourth option is also typical of an obsessive cognition. The final option is an assumption that is not typical of OCD. This is probably more typical of a depressive assumption that reinforces the core belief 'I am a failure'. As a corollary, there may be another secondary assumption – 'If I please everyone, I am considered successful'.

Freeman C and Power M. *Handbook of Evidence-based Psychotherapies: A Guide for Research and Practice,* 1st edn. WileyBlackwell, 2007, p. 146.

21. A. Covert sensitisation is a variant of aversive conditioning wherein images (e.g. of drinking situations) is paired with imaginary aversive stimuli (e.g. a scene of a person vomiting all over the place, or a scene of a person dying of alcohol-induced liver damage). It is called covert because neither the undesirable stimulus nor the aversive stimulus is actually presented except in the imagination. Sensitization refers to the intention to build up an avoidance response to the undesirable stimulus. This is based on aversion therapy.

Freeman C and Power M. *Handbook of Evidence-based Psychotherapies: A Guide for Research and Practice,* 1st edn. WileyBlackwell, 2007, p. 70.

22. B.   Parent management training was first established as a treatment programme by Gerald Patterson in the 1970s. The programme was based on the principles of learning theory, both operant theories and social learning theories, which teach parents to use positive reinforcers, like stickers, toys, or snacks to increase positive behaviour, while using time out tactics to reduce negative behaviour like temper tantrums. Focus is on one problem behaviour at a time. The parents are taught to observe the problem behaviour – the situations and timings at which it occurs. The frequency of this behaviour is usually charted to look at the progress, while abstinence from the behaviour is positively rewarded and indulgence in the behaviour is rewarded with time outs. Parents are also taught to identify behaviours that are incompatible with the 'problem' behaviour – e.g. talking nicely instead of whining. These are called 'competing' behaviours – and these are usually rewarded. Consistency in rewarding and punishing is important in this setting. This treatment is usually used in childhood disruptive disorders such as oppositional defiant disorder or conduct disorder. Shaping and chaining are operant techniques used to induce target behaviours. Approximating 'da' and 'da' to form the word 'dada' – to which the daddy hugs the child (reinforcer) is an example of shaping. Chaining is linking of more complex tasks such as wearing a pull-over shirt – this consists of a number of complex steps. Modelling is a social learning technique where a social behaviour is reinforced by society. For example a student who changes dress to fit in with a certain group of students has a strong likelihood of being accepted and thus reinforced by that group.

Koocher GP, Norcross JC and Hill SS. *Psychologists' Desk Reference.* Oxford University Press, 2005, p. 328.

23. B.   Systematic desensitization was first developed by Joseph Wolpe in the 1950s to treat phobic patients. It is based on the principles of counter-conditioning. It attempts to replace the 'fear' response to phobic stimuli with a new response (muscle relaxation) that is incompatible with fear. The first step in systematic desensitization is to train the clients in deep relaxation until they can rapidly achieve muscle relaxation when instructed to do so. The second step is to construct what is known as an 'anxiety hierarchy', in which the client's feared situations are ordered from the least to the most anxiety-provoking. Thus, for example, a person with phobia for 'cockroaches' might regard a photograph of a cockroach as only modestly threatening, but a large, rapidly moving cockroach close by as highly threatening. The client reaches a state of deep relaxation, and is then asked to imagine (or is confronted by the photograph of a cockroach) the least threatening situation in the anxiety hierarchy. The client repeatedly imagines (or is confronted by) this situation until it fails to evoke any anxiety at all, indicating that the counter-conditioning has been successful. This process is repeated while working through the levels in the anxiety hierarchy until the most anxiety-provoking situation is reached.

Gelder M, Harrison P, and Cowen P. *Shorter Oxford Textbook of Psychiatry*, 5th edn. Oxford University Press, 2006, p. 591.

24. B.   Habit reversal is a complex procedure used generally to treat tics, Tourette's syndrome and stuttering. The treatment has five components – training in becoming aware of the onset of the behaviour; monitoring the behaviour; training in initiating competing responses that are compatible with the behaviour; relaxation; and social support. Training in thought stopping is not a component of habit reversal training.

Gelder M, Harrison P, and Cowen P. *Shorter Oxford Textbook of Psychiatry,* 5th edn. Oxford University Press, 2006, p. 593.

25. D. Orgasmic reconditioning was first described by Marquis in 1970. In this treatment, the individual is asked to masturbate regularly to their troublesome deviant fantasies, but at the point of orgasmic inevitability, to switch to a desired non-deviant fantasy. As treatment progresses, the non-deviant stimulus is introduced earlier and earlier in the arousal process until masturbation is achieved without the deviant fantasy. This technique obviously is used when the behaviour or sexual preference that is of concern is not in itself dangerous or causing a public nuisance. Following the treatment, further sexual and social skills training is usually needed to ensure that the arousal to non-deviant stimuli is maintained.

Naismith J and Grant S. *Seminars in the Psychotherapies*. Gaskell, 2007, p. 165.

26. A. Massed negative practice requires the individual to deliberately perform the tic accurately and with effort for a specific amount of time during the day. In theory, this is supposed to induce conditioned inhibition or conditioned fatigue of the behaviour, which results in a decrease in the tic. This is usually employed when habit reversal techniques have not been found to be useful. The evidence for the effectiveness of this treatment is not compelling, especially when compared with habit reversal training.

Naismith J and Grant S. *Seminars in the Psychotherapies*. Gaskell, 2007, p. 168.

27. B. Token economy is based on operant conditioning theory. Their aim is to reinforce desired behaviour, while undesired behaviour is extinguished or punished. In token economy, the therapist distributes so-called tokens for occurrences of desired behaviour, e.g. brushing teeth or cleaning the room. These tokens are chips that function as secondary reinforcers. The patient can exchange the tokens for various objects (such as money or sweets) and favours (like watching television or taking a walk outside). This was widely used in the treatment of schizophrenia in the past, although most behaviour techniques are thought to be of ethical concern. Voucher-based token economy programmes are also used in substance use programmes, where 'supermarket' vouchers worth certain amounts are given to the patient as a reward for abstinence.

Freeman C and Power M. *Handbook of Evidence-based Psychotherapies: A Guide for Research and Practice*, 1st edn. WileyBlackwell, 2007, 66–67.

28. A. Positive behavioural programming was developed to concentrate solely on interventions designed to increase desired behaviours with the theoretical argument that these would then replace problem behaviours. In this case there has been differential reinforcement of a more positive activity. Functional communication training is an example of positive behaviour programming. It is based on the hypothesis that problem behaviours are usually communication needs. Individuals are taught to communicate through alternative more acceptable ways.

Freeman C and Power M. *Handbook of Evidence-based Psychotherapies: A Guide for Research and Practice*, 1st edn. WileyBlackwell, 2007, p. 199.

29. E. In a 12-month follow-up randomized controlled trial of CBT vs treatment as usual, CBT was found to be better than medical care as usual. Compared with the control group, the CBT group had significantly lower levels of hypochondriacal symptoms, beliefs, and attitudes and health-related anxiety at 12 months. They also had less impairment of social role functioning and intermediate activities of daily living. However, hypochondriacal somatic symptoms did not improve significantly. The authors of the study Barsky and Ahern explained, 'Conceptually, hypochondriacal somatic symptoms cannot simply be stripped away with symptomatic treatment, because they exist for underlying psychological and interpersonal reasons. This suggests that a realistic goal in treating hypochondriasis is amelioration of distressing fears and beliefs and improved coping, rather than the elimination of somatic symptoms per se.'

Barsky AJ and Ahern DK. Cognitive behavior therapy for hypochondriasis: a randomized, controlled trial. *Journal of the American Medical Association* 2004; **291**: 1464–1470.

30. A. Most evidence suggests that CBT specific for bulimia nervosa (CBT-BN) devised by Fairburn has a better and faster outcome than most other psychological therapies. NICE guidelines recommend a self-help programme as possible first step for treatment. CBT-BN, a specifically adapted form of CBT, is offered to adults with bulimia nervosa as an alternative. The course of treatment should be for 16–20 sessions over 4–5 months. When people with bulimia nervosa have not responded to or do not want CBT, other psychological treatments should be considered. Interpersonal psychotherapy should be considered as an alternative to CBT, but patients should be informed it takes 8–12 months to achieve results similar to CBT.

Freeman C and Power M. *Handbook of Evidence-based Psychotherapies: A Guide for Research and Practice*, 1st edn. WileyBlackwell, 2007, p. 161.

NICE. CG9 Eating disorders: full guideline. Clinical Guidelines. http://guidance.nice.org.uk/CG9/Guidance/pdf/English (accessed 8 June 2009).

31. A. NICE guidelines recommend referral to CAMHS tier 2 or 3. The first step in the management is to offer one of the following specific psychological therapies (for at least 3 months) as a first-line treatment:

- individual CBT, or
- interpersonal therapy, or
- shorter-term family therapy.

If the depression is unresponsive to the above therapies in four to six sessions a multidisciplinary review should follow. Further psychological assessment for comorbidity and further psychological and social treatments that address these should be considered. Only after these steps, is medication considered as an addition.

- For young people aged 12–18 years offer fluoxetine in addition to psychological therapy.
- For children aged 5–11 years cautiously consider the addition of fluoxetine (evidence for its effectiveness in this age group is not established).

NICE. CG28 Depression in children and young people: quick reference guide. Clinical Guidelines. http://guidance.nice.org.uk/CG28/QuickRefGuide/pdf/English (accessed 8 June 2009).

32. E. In acute treatment for depression with IPT, the problem areas can be classified as role transitions (associated with stressful life events), grief, role disputes (e.g. in marriage), or interpersonal deficits (lack of social support). Although specific stressful experiences are relevant to other IPT problem areas in the broadest sense, adjusting to stress and change in the social context requires a role transition. This might be the case in depression following the birth of a child, retirement, medical illness, divorce, etc. According to IPT, bereavement is thought to be a potential precursor of clinical depression. Development of clinical depression following a death is evidence that the normal grief process did not take place and that the individual has had an abnormal grief reaction. In such cases the work of IPT is to help the patient experience the normal grief process. A role dispute can occur in any important relationship especially the patient's relationship with his or her spouse or significant other. In interpersonal deficits, the patient's primary problem is seen as a paucity of social connections. Relationships buffer the individual against stressful life events and are essential to psychological well-being. As such, the primary goal is to enhance the level of social connection through concrete positive changes in the patient's social activities (e.g. joining a club, taking a class). Attention to social support and a positive social network is also a component of work in the other IPT problem areas.

Gabbard GO. *Textbook of Psychotherapeutic Treatments in Psychiatry*, 1st edn. American Psychiatric Publishing, 2008, p. 275.

33. C. Because guilt and low self-esteem are characteristic of depression, patients frequently blame themselves and think of themselves as 'bad' when problems arise. Although many depressed patients report these negative cognitions, the therapist does not systematically question and evaluate the automatic negative thoughts. Unlike cognitive therapists, interpersonal therapists neither employ thought records nor weigh the evidence to help patients re-evaluate negative cognitions. Instead, therapists shift blame to the illness, which often provides patients with an immediate feeling of relief. Therapists then capitalize on this transient mood improvement by encouraging patients to take positive steps towards resolving interpersonal problems.

Gabbard GO. *Textbook of Psychotherapeutic Treatments in Psychiatry*, 1st edn. American Psychiatric Publishing, 2008, p. 290.

34. B. A landmark trial in the history of antidepressant psychotherapy was the multisite NIMH Treatment of Depression Collaborative Research Program. Investigators randomly assigned 250 outpatients with major depression to receive 16 weeks of IPT, CBT, imipramine plus clinical management, or placebo pills plus clinical management. This study was the first comparison of IPT and CBT, each of which had demonstrated efficacy in separate trials, and the first trial to use treatment manuals and monitor the psychotherapeutic input of pharmacotherapists. Most patients completed at least 12 once-weekly treatment sessions or 15 weeks of therapy. Those with milder depression (defined as a score of <20 on the 17-item Hamilton Rating Scale for Depression) improved equally regardless of which treatment was used. For more severely depressed patients (those with a Ham-D score of 20), imipramine worked fastest and was most consistently superior to placebo. IPT and imipramine had comparable effects on Ham-D scores and several other outcome measures, and were superior to placebo for more severely depressed patients. CBT was not superior to placebo among the more depressed patients.

Gabbard GO. *Textbook of Psychotherapeutic Treatments in Psychiatry*, 1st edn. American Psychiatric Publishing, 2008, p. 300.

35. D. Crisis intervention originated from the work of Lindemann and Caplan. It is based on Caplan's description of four stages of coping, including emotional arousal, disorganization of behaviour, trials of alternative coping and finally exhaustion and decompensation. Crisis intervention aims primarily to deal with the first stage, so that further stages can be prevented. Hence the first step is to reduce arousal, both physiological and emotional. The approach is collaborative with family and friends. Very often this stage includes the use of medications that prevent or help reduce arousal. Along with the reduction in arousal, the patient is encouraged to focus on the current problems and encourage self-help. The second stage of crisis intervention resembles problem-solving counselling and includes the assessment of patients' problems and assets, their ability to come up with solutions and test them, and finally to consider coping mechanisms for the future if similar problems arise.

Gelder M, Harrison P, and Cowen P. *Shorter Oxford Textbook of Psychiatry*, 5th edn. Oxford University Press, 2006, Oxford. p. 586.

36. D. Marsha Linehan developed dialectical therapy for patients with borderline personality disorder who repeatedly harm themselves. The treatment uses both behavioural and cognitive methods. It is highly structured and is manual based. Therapy is intense with individual sessions, skills training in a group and access by telephone to the therapist between sessions. It is delivered by a small team of therapists and lasts for up to a year. Individual sessions have four elements: cognitive behavioural techniques including self monitoring; dialectical ways of thinking about problems – seeing causality in terms of both/and rather than either/or and the possibility of reconciling opposites; mindfulness, that is the practice of detachment from the experience; use of aphorisms, that is phrases that encapsulate the approach –e.g. people may not have caused the problems, but have to solve them anyway. Skills training sessions are provided in a group basis and telephone contacts are designed to help patients get out of crises, by using the skills learnt in the sessions.

Gelder M, Harrison P, and Cowen P. *Shorter Oxford Textbook of Psychiatry*, 5th edn. Oxford University Press, 2006p. 599.

37. C. Cohesion is the sense that the group is working together towards a common goal. This is believed to be the most important factor related to positive therapeutic effects. Group cohesion has been likened to the therapeutic alliance in dyadic treatment. In dynamic therapies, specific and non-specific elements contribute to therapeutic change. In groups, the presence of other people adds to factors present in all dyadic healing relationships. Non-specific factors are embedded in the relationships established through a consistent, accepting, non-judgemental, and supportive environment. These are all elements of a cohesive group. Groups provide a corrective emotional experience in which patients experience others (including the therapist) responding to them differently from those in their past. Members share their stories (catharsis) and feel less isolated when others have shared similar stories (universalization); they have opportunities to be helpful to others through both cognitive understanding and emotional linking (imparting information, providing feedback, and altruism). They also see others improve, which conveys hope. These elements contribute to the sense of collaboration and a willingness to adopt norms (i.e. discuss feelings about the interactions in the meeting) that further members' sense of efficacy and belonging. They contribute to an experience of support and acceptance, which may be sufficient therapeutic gain for a number of patients. Fight/flight, pairing, and dependency are Bion's basic group assumptions that lead to a negative therapeutic effect.

Tasman A, Maj M, First MB, *et al. Psychiatry*, 3rd edn. WileyBlackwell, 2007, p. 1908.

38. A. Permissiveness is the principle where members tolerate behaviour that they may not accept elsewhere. This is also helped by the members having the opportunity to be helpful to others through both cognitive understanding and emotional linking (imparting information, providing feedback, and altruism). Mutual help is the process by which members support each other and help each other to change. Imitation is the conscious emulation of one's behaviour following that of another – also called role modelling. Altruism is the process of putting another person's need ahead of one's own and in the process learning there is value in giving to others.

Gelder M, Harrison P, and Cowen P. *Shorter Oxford Textbook of Psychiatry*, 5th edn. Oxford University Press, 2006, p. 608.

Sadock BJ and Sadock VA. *Kaplan and Sadock's Synopsis of Psychiatry: Behavioral Sciences/clinical Psychiatry*, 10th edn. Lippincott Williams & Wilkins, 2007, p. 937.

39. B. Circular questioning is often used in family therapy as part of assessment. The purpose is to discover and clarify confused or conflicting views among the members of the family. Following this, a hypothesis is constructed about family functioning, which is then presented to the family, who should consider it between sessions. The family may be asked to try to behave in new ways. Paradoxical injunctions are used in couples therapy and family therapy. They are provocative statements designed to elicit a beneficial counter-response that the couple have previously resisted. Very often, this will include a prescription of the 'unwanted symptom', which the couple realize and try to give reasons why this is acceptable to the couple. Socratic questioning is a technique used in cognitive therapy. Role reversal is a technique in couples therapy which helps one partner to understand the point of view and experience of the other.

Gelder M, Harrison P, and Cowen P. *Shorter Oxford Textbook of Psychiatry*, 5th edn. Oxford University Press, 2006, p. 612.

40. C. Family therapy is mostly employed in child psychiatry settings, when problems have usually been identified in a child's behaviour, which has led the family to seek help. The aim of family therapy is to improve family functioning and so help the identified patient. The goals of family therapy include (1) improved communications; (2) improved autonomy for each member; (3) improved agreement about roles; (4) reduced conflict; (5) reduced distress in the member who is the patient. Family therapy developed from Ackerman's work on psychodynamics of family and Bateson's work on communication. Ackerman's work led to the development of psychodynamic methods of treatment, while Bateson's work led to the system's approach. Minuchin developed further the system's approach in the USA to form the structural family therapy method.

Gelder M, Harrison P, and Cowen P. *Shorter Oxford Textbook of Psychiatry*, 5th edn. Oxford University Press, 2006, p. 611.

41. A. Cognitive analytical therapy was first developed by Ryle as a brief form of therapy. The therapy is based on the principle that purposeful behaviour activity always follows a sequence. These sequences can be faulty in three ways. Traps are repetitive cycles of behaviour in which the consequence of the behaviour perpetuates it. For example a depressed student is hopeless and stops studying for his exam. He fails the exam, and feels more hopeless and depressed. Dilemmas are false choices or unduly narrowed options. For example, people who fear angry feelings may think they have to choose between placation and aggression. They choose to placate others who then take advantage of them, thus making them even angrier. Snags are the anticipation of highly negative consequences of action such that the action is never carried out and therefore never subject to a reality check.

Gelder M, Harrison P, and Cowen P. *Shorter Oxford Textbook of Psychiatry*, 5th edn. Oxford University Press, 2006, p. 601.

42. D. Collaborative empiricism is a term used in cognitive therapy to describe the therapeutic relationship with a high degree of collaboration and an experimental but pragmatic tone to the therapy. This allows the therapist to formulate hypotheses and helps the client to test the validity of the hypotheses, thus actively contributing to the client's therapy. It does not necessarily mean that the client and the therapist must agree with each other on every aspect of the therapy. In addition, the therapist need not collude with dysfunctional assumptions the client holds in order to achieve the collaboration.

Sadock BJ and Sadock VA. *Kaplan and Sadock's Synopsis of Psychiatry: Behavioral Sciences/clinical Psychiatry*, 10th edn. Lippincott Williams & Wilkins, 2007, p. 964.

43. C.   Psychodrama is a method of group psychotherapy originated by Jacob Moreno, a Viennese-born psychiatrist. In this type of psychotherapy, the personality make-up, interpersonal relationships, conflicts, and emotional problems are explored by means of special 'dramatic' methods. Therapeutic dramatization of emotional problems includes the 'protagonist' or patient, the person who acts out his/her problems. The enactment is carried out with the help of 'auxiliary egos', people who enact varying aspects of the patient. The therapist takes up the role of the 'director' and guides those in the drama towards the acquisition of insight. Situations are chosen by the protagonist – this usually focuses on any special area of functioning or symptoms. The auxiliary ego takes on the role of other significant people in the protagonist's life. The therapist directs the situations, and the group can comment on various ways in which the protagonist deals with the situation he/she is in. Techniques to advance the therapeutic process and to increase productivity and creativity include the soliloquy (a recital of overt and hidden thoughts and feelings), role reversal (the exchange of the patient's role for the role of a significant person), the double (an auxiliary ego acting as the patient), the multiple double (several egos acting as the patient did on varying occasions), and the mirror technique (an ego imitating the patient and speaking for him or her). Other techniques include the use of hypnosis and psychoactive drugs to modify the acting behaviour in various ways.

Sadock BJ and Sadock VA. *Kaplan and Sadock's Synopsis of Psychiatry: Behavioral Sciences/clinical Psychiatry*, 10th edn. Lippincott Williams & Wilkins, 2007, p. 939.

44. B.   This is called applied tension. Unlike those with other specific phobias who show an increase in sympathetic output on exposure to phobic stimuli, patients with blood–injury–injection phobia show a unique, biphasic response. The first phase is associated with increased heart rate and blood pressure. In the second phase, however, the blood pressure suddenly falls and the patient faints. To treat the problem, patients are shown a series of slides that are provocative (e.g. mutilated bodies). They are trained to identify early-warning signs of fainting, such as queasiness, cold sweats, or dizziness. They also learn how to apply the learned muscle tension response quickly, contingent on these warning signs. Patients can also perform applied tension while donating blood or watching a surgical operation. The technique of isometric tension raises blood pressure, which prevents fainting.

Sadock BJ and Sadock VA. *Kaplan and Sadock's Synopsis of Psychiatry: Behavioral Sciences/clinical Psychiatry*, 10th edn. Lippincott Williams & Wilkins, 2007, p. 952.

45. B.   The acronym FRAMES captures the essence of a number of interventions commonly used under the terms 'brief intervention'. These are interventions that cover a range from one 5-minute interaction to several 45-minute sessions. The major positive studies discussed in this section typically consist of one interaction lasting between 5 and 20 minutes, sometimes with one brief follow-up contact. The acronym FRAMES stands for: feedback: about personal risk or impairment; responsibility: emphasis on personal responsibility for change; advice: to cut down or abstain if indicated because of severe dependence or harm; menu: of alternative options for changing drinking pattern and, jointly with the patient, setting a target; intermediate goals of reduction can be a start; empathic interviewing: listening reflectively without cajoling or confronting; exploring with patients the reasons for change as they see their situation; self-efficacy: an interviewing style that enhances people's belief in their ability to change. 'Rolling with resistance' is a part of Miller and Rollnick's motivational interviewing.

SIGN guidelines No: 74; The management of harmful drinking and alcohol dependence in primary care. http://www.sign.ac.uk/guidelines/fulltext/74/index.html

46. B.   Treatment of borderline personality disorder is organized around the level of the disorder, with each level corresponding to one of four stages of treatment with specific goals that are targeted towards core deficits seen in these patients.

Stage I: In the first stage of treatment, the therapist seeks to increase behavioural control through helping patients attain basic capacities. This is targeted towards the severe 'behavioural dyscontrol' exhibited by the patient.

Stage II: The second stage targets 'quiet desperation'. The intent in this stage is to facilitate emotional experiencing through reducing post-traumatic stress and blocking dissociation. The principal goal of this stage is to block avoidance of emotions and the environmental cues associated with them. In this stage, patients are helped to experience their feelings without avoiding life or experiencing symptoms of post-traumatic stress disorder.

Stage III: The third stage is targeted towards 'problematic patterns in living'. The goal of this stage is to achieve 'ordinary happiness and unhappiness' through increasing self-respect and working on problems with relationships and career choices.

Stage IV: The fourth and final stage is directed towards 'incompleteness'. The goal of the last stage is to develop the patient's capacity for sustained experience of contentment, connection, and freedom.

Gabbard GO. *Textbook of Psychotherapeutic Treatments in Psychiatry*, 1st edn. American Psychiatric Publishing, 2008, p. 736.

47. A.   The NICE recommends 'Watchful waiting' when symptoms are mild and have been present for less than 4 weeks after the trauma, with a follow-up contact within 1 month. NICE specifically asks therapists and clinicians not to routinely offer brief, single-session interventions (debriefing) that focus on the traumatic incident to that individual alone. Where symptoms are present for less than 3 months (as in the case with Rachel), NICE specifically recommends trauma-focused CBT (usually on an individual outpatient basis. Trauma-focused CBT is also recommended for people with 'severe' symptoms or 'severe' PTSD within 1 month. NICE recommends 8–12 weekly sessions of trauma-focused CBT, each session delivered by the same person and lasting around 90 minutes during which trauma is discussed. NICE advises against the use of non-directed therapies such as relaxation training. Where symptoms are milder and have lasted for more than 3 months, NICE recommends either trauma-focused CBT or EMDR. In addition to psychological treatments, NICE also recommends specific pharmacological interventions.

NICE. Clinical Guideline 26: Post-traumatic stress disorder (PTSD): the management of PTSD in adults and children in primary and secondary care. www.nice.org.uk/CG026NICEguideline

48. B. Biofeedback is the process where certain physiological parameters of an individual are recorded and displayed. It is usually used in combination with relaxation. This involves the recording of small changes in the physiological levels (induced by relaxation) of the feedback parameter. The display can be visual or auditory. Patients are instructed to change the levels of the physiological parameter, using the feedback from the display. It is based on the idea that the autonomic nervous system can come under voluntary control through operant conditioning. The feedback instrument used depends on the patient and the specific problem. The most effective instruments are the electromyogram (EMG), which measures the electrical potentials of muscle fibres; the electroencephalogram (EEG), which measures alpha waves that occur in relaxed states; the galvanic skin response (GSR) gauge, which shows decreased skin conductivity during a relaxed state; and the thermistor, which measures skin temperature (which drops during tension because of peripheral vasoconstriction). For example, in the treatment of bruxism, an EMG electrode is attached to the masseter muscle. The EMG emits a loud tone when the muscle is contracted and a low tone when at rest. Patients can learn to alter the tone to indicate relaxation. Patients receive feedback about the masseter muscle, the tone reinforces the learning, and the condition ameliorates.

Sadock BJ and Sadock VA. *Kaplan and Sadock's Synopsis of Psychiatry: Behavioral Sciences/clinical Psychiatry*, 10th edn. Lippincott Williams & Wilkins, 2007, p. 950.

49. B. Schemas determine our perceptions, assimilations, and actions upon the externally received information. These are developed through early experiences in childhood and formative influences thereafter. According to Beck, these are deeper cognitive structures than the negative automatic thoughts that are readily observable in clients undergoing cognitive behavioural therapy. Everyone interacts with the external world by utilizing his/her set of schemas. Most of these are simple schemas that do not contribute to any psychopathology. So schemas are conditional rules ('if–then statements') while the others are core beliefs about oneself ('I am good-looking', 'I cannot write a poem', etc). Clients requiring CBT often have a cluster of maladaptive schemas that perpetuate depression or anxiety state.

Kaplan HI. *Kaplan and Sadock's Comprehensive Textbook of Psychiatry*, 8th edn. Lippincott Williams & Wilkins, 2004. p. 2516.

50. C. Clients with generalized anxiety often have an attentional bias that sensitizes them to respond to potentially threatening stimuli in the environment. Such attentional biases towards threatening information are also noted in individuals with high trait anxiety and may play an important role in the development of clinical anxiety disorders and maintenance of anxiety. Experimentally, dot probe tasks have been used to demonstrate such biases. Clients with depression often underestimate positive aspects of life, e.g. downplaying positive feedback but continuing with a sense of failure and hopelessness. They might also exhibit absolute thinking favouring negative themes – this is termed as black and white thinking.

Koster EH, Crombez G, Verschuere B, *et al.*, Attention to threat in anxiety-prone individuals: mechanisms underlying attentional bias. *Cognitive Therapy and Research* **30**: 635–643.

1. **A study is evaluating the effect of agomelatine on postnatal depression at a mother and baby unit. Which one of the following should be considered when assessing the internal validity of this study?**

    A. Benefits of agomelatine in major depression outside the postpartum period
    B. The degree to which the subjects adhered to the study protocol
    C. The cost of using agomelatine compared with standard care
    D. Consistency of the reported outcome in comparison with previous studies
    E. Benefits of agomelatine in postpartum depression when used at an outpatient service

2. **A new clinician-administered test for assessing suicidal risk is studied in a prison population in Canada, where a high suicide rate of 1 in 25 has been recorded. Which of the following indicate that this test is NOT suitable for your clinical population?**

    A. The positive predictive value is 80%
    B. The likelihood ratio for a positive test is 14
    C. The prevalence of suicide in your clinical sample is 1 in 890
    D. The inter-rater reliability (kappa) of the test is 0.8
    E. The literacy rate of the prison population is very low but comparable with your clinical sample

3. **A new rating scale being evaluated for anxiety has a sensitivity of 80% and specificity of 90% against the standard ICD-10 diagnosis. The likelihood ratio of a positive result is**

    A. Nearly 2
    B. Nearly 0.2
    C. 0.08
    D. 8
    E. 0.5

4.   A pharmaceutical company developed a new antidepressant 'X'. They
     conducted a randomized double-blind placebo controlled trial of the drug.
     The study had two arms: an active medication arm and a placebo arm.
     Each arm had 100 subjects. Over a 4-week period, a 50% drop in Hamilton
     depression scale (HAMD) scores were seen in 40 subjects in the active
     medication arm, while a similar drop was seen only in 20 subjects in the
     placebo arm. What is the number needed to treat (NNT) from this trial for
     the new antidepressant?

     A. 1
     B. 2
     C. 3
     D. 4
     E. 5

5.   During the same placebo controlled trial described in question 4, 20% of
     people on X developed active suicidal ideas, while only 10% of patients on
     placebo developed the same side-effect. What is the number needed to
     harm (NNH) associated with the suicidal ideas from the trial data?

     A. 5
     B. 10
     C. 15
     D. 20
     E. 25

6.   The prevalence of depression in patients with mild cognitive impairment
     is 10%. On applying a depression rating scale with the likelihood ratio of a
     positive test (LR+) equal to 10, a patient with mild cognitive impairment
     becomes test positive. The probability that this patient is depressed is equal
     to

     A. 15%
     B. 32%
     C. 52%
     D. 85%
     E. 100%

7.   A multi-centre double blind pragmatic randomized controlled trial (RCT)
     reported remission rates for depression of 65% for fluoxetine and 60% for
     dosulepin. The number of patients that must receive fluoxetine for one
     patient to achieve the demonstrated beneficial effect is

     A. 60
     B. 20
     C. 15
     D. 10
     E. 5

8. In a randomized double-blind trial two groups of hospitalized depressed patients treated with selective serotonin reuptake inhibitors (SSRIs) are evaluated for beneficial effects on insomnia of trazodone vs temazepam. Which of the following is NOT an important factor when evaluating the internal validity of results obtained from the above study?

    A. Baseline differences in antidepressant therapy between the two groups
    B. The method used to randomize the sample
    C. Setting in which the study takes place
    D. Sensitivity of the insomnia scale to pick up changes in severity
    E. Inclusion of the data in final analysis from patients who have dropped out

9. While adapting the results of an RCT into clinical practice, a clinician wants to calculate the new NNT values for his own clinical population using the results of the RCT. Apart from the reported RCT which of the following is needed to carry out the calculation of the new NNT?

    A. The expected rate of spontaneous resolution of the treated condition in the clinical population
    B. The size of the clinical population
    C. The case fatality rate for the treated condition in the clinical population
    D. Lifetime prevalence of the disease in the clinical population
    E. All of the above

10 In an attempt to ensure equivalent distribution of potential effect-modifying factors in treating refractory depression, a researcher weighs the imbalance that might be caused whenever an individual patient enters one of the two arms of the study. Every patient is assigned to the group where the least amount of imbalance will be caused. This method is called

    A. Stratification
    B. Matching
    C. Minimization
    D. Randomization
    E. Systematic sampling

11. The effectiveness of an intervention is measured by using pragmatic trials. Which trial design is normally employed when carrying out a pragmatic trial?

    A. RCT
    B. Meta analysis
    C. Systematic review
    D. Cohort study
    E. Case series

12. **The probability of detecting the magnitude of a treatment effect from a study when such an effect actually exists is called**

    A. Validity
    B. Precision
    C. Accuracy
    D. Power
    E. Yield

13. **Power is the ability of a study to detect an effect that truly exists. Power can also be defined as**

    A. Probability of avoiding type 1 error
    B. Probability of committing type 1 error
    C. Probability of committing type 2 error
    D. Probability of detecting a type 2 error
    E. Probability of avoiding type 2 error

14. **A new diagnostic test detects 60 out of 100 schizophrenia patients correctly. It does not wrongly diagnose anyone in a sample of 100 controls. The positive predictive value of this test is**

    A. 50%
    B. 60%
    C. 40%
    D. 100%
    E. 0%

15. **A new diagnostic test detects 60 out of 100 schizophrenia patients correctly. It does not wrongly diagnose anyone in a sample of 100 controls. How sensitive is this test in detecting schizophrenia?**

    A. 60%
    B. 40%
    C. 100%
    D. 90%
    E. 0%

16. **A new diagnostic test detects 60 out of 100 schizophrenia patients correctly. It does not wrongly diagnose anyone in a sample of 100 controls. How accurate is this test in detecting schizophrenia?**

    A. 100%
    B. 80%
    C. 60%
    D. 40%
    E. 70%

17. **A new diagnostic test detects 60 out of 100 schizophrenia patients correctly. It does not wrongly diagnose anyone in a sample of 100 controls. What are the chances that the text will turn negative in your next patient with schizophrenia?**

    A. 100%
    B. 70%
    C. 60%
    D. 40%
    E. 30%

18. **Which of the following properties of a screening test increases with increasing disease prevalence in the population?**

    A. Negative predictive value
    B. Sensitivity
    C. Specificity
    D. Accuracy
    E. Positive predictive value

19. **Two observers are rating MRI scans for the presence or absence of white matter hyperintensities. On a particular day from the records, they are observed to have an agreement of 78%. If they could be expected to agree 50% of the time, even if the process of detecting hyperintensities is by pure chance, then the value of kappa statistics is given by**

    A. 50%
    B. 44%
    C. 56%
    D. 78%
    E. 22%

20. **The number of days that a series of five patients had to wait before starting cognitive behavioural therapy (CBT) at a psychotherapy unit is as follows: 12, 12, 14, 16, and 21. The median waiting time to get CBT is**

    A. 15 days
    B. 12 days
    C. 14 days
    D. 21 days
    E. 13 days

21. **The number of days that a series of five patients had to wait before starting CBT at a psychotherapy unit is as follows: 12, 12, 14, 16, and 21. The mean waiting time to get CBT is**

    A. 15 days
    B. 12 days
    C. 14 days
    D. 21 days
    E. 13 days

22. The most clinically useful measure that helps to inform the likelihood of having a disease in a patient with positive results from a diagnostic test is

    A. Accuracy
    B. Positive predictive value
    C. Sensitivity
    D. Specificity
    E. Reliability

23. Zarkin et al., 2008 reported the cost-effectiveness comparison of naltrexone and placebo in alcohol abstinence. The mean effectiveness measured as percentage days of abstinence was nearly 80% for naltrexone group while it was 73% for the placebo group. The mean cost incurred for the placebo group was $400 per patient. The naltrexone group incurred a cost of 680 per patient. How much additional cost needs to be spent per patient for each percentage point increase in total days of abstinence when using naltrexone compared with placebo?

    A. $40
    B. $50
    C. $7
    D. $500
    E. $2

24. Two continuous variables A and B are found to be correlated in a non-linear fashion. All of the following can be considered as suitable statistical techniques for examining this relationship except

    A. Curvilinear regression
    B. Logistic regression
    C. Multiple linear regression
    D. Polynomial regression
    E. Exponential regression

25. A drug representative presents data on a new trial. The data show that drug A prevents annual hospitalization in 20% more dementia patients than placebo. You are very impressed but your consultant wants to know how many patients you need to treat to prevent one hospitalization. The correct answer is

    A. 20
    B. 5
    C. 80
    D. 1
    E. 100

26. **A new study attempts to evaluate the benefits of regular exercise in preventing depression compared with unmodified lifestyle in a sample of 80 healthy elderly men. Which of the following is not possible in such a study design?**
   A. Randomized trial
   B. Allocation concealed trial
   C. Prospective trial
   D. Double-blinded trial
   E. Controlled trial

27. **When searching medical databases, the term MeSH refers to**
   A. Software that distributes all indexed articles
   B. A keyword that will retrieve all published articles by an author
   C. A thesaurus of medical subject headings
   D. A keyword that stops ongoing search process
   E. A database of mental health and social care topics

28. **Which of the following is strictly correct about a single-blind study design?**
   A. Only the patients, but not the researchers, do not know whether placebo or active drug is being administered
   B. Only the researchers, but not the patients, do not know whether placebo or active drug is being administered
   C. Both the patient and researchers do not know the treatment given
   D. Only one group of the trial subjects is kept unaware of the treatment status
   E. Either the patients or the researchers do not know whether placebo or active drug is administered

29. **Which one of the following correctly describes a crossover trial?**
   A. Halfway through the treatment phase, the subjects from both arms interchange randomly
   B. Each subject receives both intervention and control with a washout period in between
   C. Controls from one trial are shared with another trial where a different drug is evaluated simultaneously
   D. The trial permits investigation of the effect of more than one independent variable on the clinical outcome
   E. None of the above

30. **A study evaluates the effect of various psychological interventions on bulimia. This study could be termed as a factorial design if**
   A. Halfway through the treatment phase, the subjects from two arms interchange randomly
   B. Each subject receives both intervention and control with a washout period in between
   C. Controls from one trial are shared with another trial where a totally different psychotherapy is evaluated simultaneously
   D. The trial permits investigation of the effect of more than one psychotherapy, both separately and combined, on the clinical outcome.
   E. None of the above

31. **A 2 × 2 contingency table is constructed to analyse the primary outcome data of a trial. The degrees of freedom to use chi-square statistics is**
    A. 1
    B. 2
    C. 3
    D. 4
    E. −4

32. **Which one of the following is correctly matched with the most suitable study method?**
    A. Diagnostic test: case–control study
    B. Prognosis: prospective cohort study
    C. Therapy: cross-sectional survey
    D. Aetiology: case–series study
    E. Epidemiology: RCT.

33. **Which of the following characters of a pragmatic RCT distinguishes it from an explanatory RCT?**
    A. Pseudo-randomization is practised in pragmatic trials
    B. Type 1 error level is set to be higher in pragmatic trials
    C. Descriptive rather than inferential statistics are used to report the outcome of pragmatic trials
    D. Higher generalizability is achieved in pragmatic trials
    E. Strict exclusion of patients with comorbid conditions is seen in pragmatic trials

34. **Which one of the following statement with respect to bias is false?**
    A. Bias is a systematic error
    B. Bias cannot be controlled for during the analysis stage of a trial
    C. The presence of bias always overestimates the final effect
    D. Blinding reduces measurement bias
    E. Randomization reduces selection bias

35. **Which one of the following is NOT a major disadvantage of a double blind, well-concealed RCT design?**
    A. Very expensive to carry out
    B. May become time consuming
    C. Experimental results may not translate to clinical samples
    D. Randomization may be unethical and not possible in certain cases
    E. Introduction of recall bias

36. **The last observation carried forward (LOCF) method is not suitable for processing the data for which of the following RCTs with intention to treat analysis?**
    A. Benzodiazepines for anxiety
    B. SSRIs for depression
    C. Venlafaxine for generalized anxiety disorder
    D. Memantine for Alzheimer's disease
    E. Risperidone for bipolar disorder

37. **All of the following measures can be used to decrease the heterogeneity in a meta-analysis except**
    A. Transformation of the outcome variable in question
    B. Employing meta regression analysis
    C. Using a random effects model
    D. Doing a subgroup analysis
    E. Including data from smaller unpublished studies

38. **Both odds ratios and relative risk are often used as outcome measures in published studies. Which of the following statement is true regarding these measures?**
    A. The odds ratio cannot be calculated in cohort studies
    B. Incidence rate is required to calculate the odds ratio
    C. Relative risk cannot be calculated for case–control studies
    D. If the outcome of interest is very common, the odds ratio approximates relative risk
    E. The odds ratio cannot be used to study dichotomous outcomes

39. **Which one of the following clinical question can be correctly addressed by a case–control design?**
    A. Is it effective to use hyoscine patches in treating clozapine-induced hypersalivation?
    B. How many inpatients in wards for elderly people suffer from untreated hypercholesterolaemia at any given time?
    C. How rapidly will lithium discontinuation produce relapse of schizoaffective disorder?
    D. Are we at local community team compliant with the NICE guidelines for prescribing antipsychotics?
    E. Do patients with depression have more academic examination failures than their healthy siblings?

40. A 50-year-old man sustained significant memory loss following near-fatal carbon monoxide poisoning. Following discussion he agreed to take part in a double-blinded trial of donepezil vs placebo administered in six separate 4-week modules with a 2-week washout period in between. Neuropsychological measures were obtained at regular pre-planned intervals to monitor changes. He was the sole subject on the trial and the randomization sequence was generated and maintained by the pharmacy. This study design could be best described as

    A. Uncontrolled trial
    B. N-of-1 trial
    C. Crossover RCT
    D. Pragmatic RCT
    E. Naturalistic observational study

41. While conducting a systematic review, publication bias could be determined using which of the following methods?

    A. Funnel plot
    B. Galbraith plot
    C. Failsafe N
    D. Soliciting and comparing published vs. unpublished data
    E. All of the above

42. In a RCT the randomization sequence is protected before and until the randomization is completed. This is known as

    A. Concealment
    B. Double blinding
    C. Matching
    D. Masking
    E. Trial independence

43. Data collected for a study on antidepressant efficacy show the outcome as observations of the number of days needed to achieve remission. The standard deviation for such observations will be measured in which of the following units?

    A. No units
    B. Days
    C. Square root of days
    D. Days square
    E. Person-years

44. **In a study presenting outcome in terms of median days of hospital admission, the collected data show many observations substantially higher than the median. Which one of the following is correct regarding the above study?**

   A. The results are negatively skewed
   B. Mean = median = mode
   C. The results are not skewed
   D. Mean > median
   E. Mode = median

45. **A trial is conducted to evaluate the efficacy of lamotrigine in patients with symptoms of recurrent depersonalization. While calculating the number of patients needed in the trial to demonstrate a meaningful effect, α level is set at 0.05. Which of the following is true regarding alpha (α)?**

   A. It is the probability of a type 2 error
   B. It is the threshold for defining clinical significance
   C. If $\alpha = 0.05$, there is a 5% chance that the null hypothesis is rejected wrongly
   D. If $\alpha = 0.05$, then 5% of treated subjects will show absence of treatment effect.
   E. None of the above

46. **Which of the following is an agreed method of assessing the quality of conducting and reporting systematic reviews and meta-analyses?**

   A. ASSERT
   B. CONSORT
   C. QUOROM
   D. SIGN
   E. NICE

47. **All of the following methods are used to assess heterogeneity in a meta-analysis except**

   A. Q statistic
   B. I squared statistic
   C. Galbraith plot
   D. L'Abbé plot
   E. Paired t statistics

48. **Which one of the following types of data can have potentially infinite number of values?**

   A. Continuous
   B. Categorical
   C. Nominal
   D. Ordinal
   E. Binary

49. **A multi-centre RCT was conducted with strict inclusion criteria. Which one of the following properties of the study is most likely to be affected by the stringent inclusion criteria?**
    A. Generalizability of results
    B. Precision of results
    C. Accuracy of the results
    D. Statistical significance of the results
    E. All of the above

50. **A researcher is interested in studying whether maternal smoking increases the risk of school refusal in children. Which one of the following is the correct null hypothesis for the above research question?**
    A. School refusal increases the risk of maternal smoking
    B. Maternal smoking decreases the risk of school refusal
    C. Maternal smoking does not increase the risk of school refusal
    D. Maternal smoking increases the risk of school refusal
    E. None of the above

51. **From the following example, the most important methodological challenge while conducting a cohort study is**
    A. Statistical analysis of the results
    B. Randomization of the cohorts
    C. Identifying those who develop the outcome
    D. Identifying a suitable comparison group
    E. Concealment of cohort allocation

52. **In a study investigating the mean cholesterol levels in 36 patients taking olanzapine, the mean was found to be 262 mg/dL. The standard deviation of this observation was 15 mg/dL. The 95% confidence interval for this observation is are**
    A. 232–292 mg/dL
    B. 247–277 mg/dL
    C. 259.5–264.5 mg/dL
    D. 257–267 mg/dL
    E. 226–298 mg/dL

53. **In a normal distribution curve, 99% of observations will fall within which of the following values of standard deviation (SD)?**
    A. −2 SD to +2 SD
    B. −3 SD to +3 SD
    C. −1 SD to +2 SD
    D. −1 SD to +1 SD
    E. +1 SD to +3SD

54. **Confidence intervals are used to describe the range of uncertainty around the estimated value of an outcome from the sample studied. Which of the following statements about confidence intervals is incorrect?**

    A. Sample size is used in calculating confidence intervals
    B. It includes a range of values above and below the point estimate
    C. If the confidence interval includes a null treatment effect, the null hypothesis can be rejected
    D. 95% confidence interval is often used in clinical studies
    E. When the estimated outcome is a ratio, a positive treatment effect is shown by confidence intervals remaining above one.

55. **A clinical researcher is examining the incidence of akathisia in two groups of patients. One group (n = 35) has been prescribed benzodiazepine for use as required while the other group (n = 35) is free from any benzodiazepine exposure. The outcome is measured as proportion of patients who develop akathisia in a dichotomous scale. Akathisia develops in 10 patients without benzodiazepines and in 20 patients with benzodiazepines. Which of the following statistical tests is best suited to analyse the statistical significance of the difference between the two groups?**

    A. Chi square test
    B. Paired t test
    C. Multiple regression analysis
    D. Wilcoxon rank sum test
    E. Pearson coefficient test

56. **Considering normal distribution, which one of the following statements is incorrect?**

    A. It is a continuous distribution
    B. It is symmetrical in shape
    C. The mean, median, and mode are identical
    D. The shape of the distribution depends on the number of observations made
    E. Both tails of the distribution extend to infinity

57. **In descriptive statistics, which of the following is the most widely used measure of dispersion of a frequency distribution?**

    A. Range
    B. Median
    C. Standard deviation
    D. Variance
    E. p Value

58. **In qualitative research which of the following refers to modifying the research methods and hypothesis as and while one conducts the research?**

    A. Triangulation
    B. Iterative approach
    C. Theoretical sampling
    D. Content analysis
    E. Deductive approach

59. **Systolic blood pressure is known to be normally distributed across the population with a mean of 120 mmHg and standard deviation of 10 mmHg. How many out of 100 patients in a population will have systolic blood pressure between 120 and 130 mmHg?**

    A. 68
    B. 97
    C. 48
    D. 17
    E. 34

60. **In which of the following situations is intention to treat analysis deliberately not attempted even if there are significant numbers of drop-outs?**

    A. A study that analyses the efficacy of an intervention itself
    B. A study that analyses the effectiveness of providing an intervention
    C. A study that compares two interventions for economic efficiency
    D. A study that compares an established standard treatment against a new treatment with the view of replacing the standard
    E. None of the above

61. **A 24-week RCT of memantine in moderate–severe Alzheimer's dementia was reported. The investigators recruited 126 subjects for the memantine arm and 126 for the placebo arm, out of which 100 in the memantine group and 100 in the placebo group completed the study. Using a categorical measure of treatment response it was shown that 40% of the patients in the memantine group responded while only 20% in placebo group showed a response. Calculate the relative risk reduction of using memantine**

    A. 20
    B. 5
    C. 2
    D. 1
    E. 10

62. **Using the above study results calculate the number needed to treat (NNT) for patients receiving memantine compared with placebo**

    A. 20
    B. 5
    C. 2
    D. 10
    E. 7

63. **If the above study used a per protocol analysis of primary outcome, the odds ratio of having a response is**

    A. 2.7
    B. 7.2
    C. 0.16
    D. 6
    E. 0.37

64. **Which one of the following measures is used in correlation analysis for non-parametric data?**

    A. Kappa statistics
    B. Pearson's correlation
    C. Spearman's correlation
    D. Cohen's d
    E. Cronbach's alpha

65. **Parametric statistical methods make assumptions, which when satisfied make the final estimate precise and accurate. Which of the following is one such parametric assumption?**

    A. The distribution of observations in the population is not known
    B. The variance of the compared samples are homogeneous
    C. The analysed variables are categorical measures
    D. Outliers are unequally distributed
    E. The sample size is at least 2% of the size of target population

66. **In a study comparing drug A and a placebo control, 20 out of 200 patients taking drug A die after 3 years. Twenty-five out of 225 patients taking the placebo die after 3 years. If death is the outcome of interest, the control event rate is given by**

    A. 25/225
    B. 20/200
    C. (25 − 20)/200
    D. (25 − 20)/225
    E. 25

67. **In an RCT comparing the effect of exposure therapy versus cognitive restructuring, follow-up was carried out at 6, 11, 24, and 36 weeks. At weeks 6 and 11, after rating the patient, the outcome assessors tried to guess the treatment condition. Correctness of guesses did not differ significantly from that expected by chance. This was an attempt to demonstrate which of the following?**

    A. Adequacy of randomization
    B. Concealment of allocation
    C. Blindness of assessor
    D. Blindness of patient
    E. Matching of two groups

68. **If the sample size is sufficiently large, mean values of repeated observations follow normal distribution irrespective of the distribution of original data in the population. This is known as**
    A. Bayesian theorem
    B. Central limit theorem
    C. Bonferroni correction
    D. Transformation theorem
    E. Independent observations theorem

69. **The validity of a new instrument is compared with an external criterion. A conceptually related external criterion is identified to occur sometime in the future. If the correlation between current scores obtained using the instrument and the future expected outcome is studied, this is called**
    A. Concurrent validity
    B. Incremental validity
    C. Predictive validity
    D. Inter-rater reliability
    E. Internal consistency

70–82 **A recent study conducted in a palliative care unit assessed the use of a two-item questionnaire to screen for the presence of depression. Given below is the table which compares the result of the screen to the gold standard (DSM-IV) diagnosis. In relation to this table, answer questions 70–82**

Overall screen (2 questions)	Actual case of major depressive disorder (DSM-IV)		Total
	Depressed	Not depressed	
Yes	39	40	79
No	4	84	88
Total	43	124	167

Payne A, Barry S, Creedon B, *et al.* Sensitivity and specificity of a two-question screening tool for depression in a specialist palliative care unit *Palliatlve Medicine* 2007; **21**: 193.

70. **The sensitivity of the overall screen using both items is approximately**
    A. 100%
    B. 25%
    C. 67%
    D. 76%
    E. 91%

71. **The specificity of the overall screen is approximately**
    A. 67%
    B. 95%
    C. 38%
    D. 25%
    E. 91%

72. The predictive power of a positive test using the overall screen is
    A. 49%
    B. 91%
    C. 67%
    D. 25%
    E. 95%

73. The predictive power of a negative test using the overall two-item screen is given by
    A. 49%
    B. 91%
    C. 67%
    D. 25%
    E. 95%

74. The pretest probability of the overall two-item screen is
    A. 49%
    B. 91%
    C. 67%
    D. 25%
    E. 95%

75. The likelihood ratio of a positive test for the overall two-item screen is
    A. 2.8
    B. 4.8
    C. 6.8
    D. 8.8
    E. 10.8

76. The likelihood ratio of a negative test (LR–) for the overall two-item screen is
    A. 0.14
    B. 0.34
    C. 0.54
    D. 0.74
    E. 0.94

77. **Using the nomogram below, calculate the post-test probability of a positive test when using the two-item depression screening test in the palliative care unit using the figures indicated at the beginning of Question 70.**

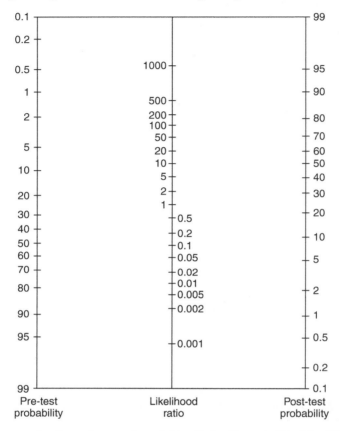

Fagan TJ. Nomogram for Bayes theorem (letter). *New England Journal of Medicine* 1975; **293**: 257.

A. 1
B. 2
C. 4
D. 10
E. 50

78. **Using the nomogram in Question 77, calculate the post-test probability of a negative test when using the two-item depression screening test in the palliative care unit**

A. 1
B. 4
C. 10
D. 50
E. 80

79. What is the false positive rate for the overall 2-items screening test?

A. 32%

B. 9%

C. 90%

D. 67%

E. 25%

80. What is the false negative rate for the overall two-item screening test?

A. 32%

B. 9%

C. 90%

D. 67%

E. 25%

81. Taking into consideration the above screening test, we randomly pick 1000 people from the general population. Considering the prevalence of a major depressive disorder using DSM-IV in the general population as 10%, calculate the positive predictive value of the 2-item screening test in the population?

A. 49%

B. 91%

C. 67%

D. 31%

E. 95%

82. Taking into consideration the above screening test, we randomly pick 1000 people from the general population. Considering the prevalence of a major depressive disorder in the general population using DSM-IV as 10%, calculate the new negative predictive value of the two-item screening test in the population?

A. 49%

B. 91%

C. 67%

D. 30%

E. 98%

83–86. The table below shows the adverse events reported during an RCT on sertraline for the prevention of relapse in detoxicated alcohol-dependent patients with a comorbid depressive disorder. Answer Questions 83–86 based on the data presented in the table

Adverse event	Placebo (n = 39)	Sertraline (n = 44)	Total (N = 83)
Headache	11	12	23
Influenza-like symptoms	6	6	12
Dizziness	5	5	10
Dyspepsia	2	6	8
Diarrhoea	3	4	7
Nausea	3	4	7

Gual AM, Balcells MM, Torres MM, et al. Sertraline for the prevention of relapse in detoxicated alcohol dependent patients with a comorbid depressive disorder: a randomized controlled trial. *Alcohol Alcohol* 2003; **38**: 619–625.

83. **What proportion of patients develops dyspepsia after exposure to the sertraline?**

    A. 13.6%
    B. 5%
    C. 8.6%
    D. 63.2%
    E. 90.2%

84. **What proportion of dyspepsia will be eliminated if sertraline was not administered?**

    A. 13.6%
    B. 5%
    C. 8.6%
    D. 63.2%
    E. 90.2%

85. **How many times is a person on sertraline more likely to develop dyspepsia than a person on placebo?**

    A. 1.7
    B. 2.7
    C. 3.7
    D. 4.7
    E. 5.7

86. How many times are the odds of being dyspeptic on sertraline higher than the odds of being dyspeptic on placebo?

    A. 1.9
    B. 2.9
    C. 3.9
    D. 4.9
    E. 5.9

87–91. The finding of a hypothetical cost-effectiveness analysis of a new model of psychotherapy in depression is shown in the table below

Treatment	Costs	Effect (number of depression-free weeks)
Antidepressants	£ 5,000	45 weeks
Psychotherapy (new treatment)	£ 10,000	50 weeks

87. Calculate the average cost-effectiveness ratio (ACER) for the new treatment?

    A. £200/week
    B. £100/week
    C. £50/week
    D. £111/week
    E. £20/week

88. Calculate the incremental cost-effectiveness ratio (ICER) for the new treatment

    A. £1000 per additional depression-free week
    B. £200 per additional depression-free week
    C. £111 per additional depression-free week
    D. £89 per additional depression-free week
    E. £600 per additional depression-free week

89. What is the incremental net benefit (INB) if the health commissioners are willing to pay around £1500 per additional depression free week?

    A. £500
    B. £1000
    C. £2500
    D. 5 weeks
    E. 1 week

90. **After critically appraising the above cost-effectiveness analysis paper, managers of an NHS foundation trust decide to choose psychotherapy over antidepressants as the first-line management for depression. Which of the following statements best defines the opportunity costs?**
    A. The original cost incurred while providing psychotherapy as the first choice treatment
    B. The cost of providing psychotherapy instead of prescribing antidepressant drugs for depression
    C. The apparent cost of not providing antidepressants as the first choice of treatment.
    D. The cost of the using antidepressants in the absence of psychotherapy for depression.
    E. The cost of conducting this trial in order to make treatment recommendations

91. **The given cost-effectiveness acceptability curve (CEAC) is drawn using the data from the hypothetical study on treatment of depression. What is the probability of cost-effectiveness if the society is willing to pay £150 for every depression-free day?**

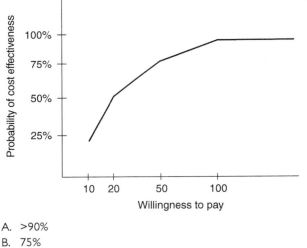

    A. >90%
    B. 75%
    C. 50%
    D. 25%
    E. <10%

92–96. A new 12-point scale with scores from 1 to 12 (1 being not depressed and 12 being the highest degree of depression) was developed to screen for depression in a population of patients with dementia. The scale was tested against the gold standard of DSM-IV in a small study. The neurologists using the test wanted a score that would identify a depressed person from a non-depressed based on this instrument. A statistician involved in the development of this instrument mailed the following graph to the neurologists. Answer Questions 96–99 based on the graph below.

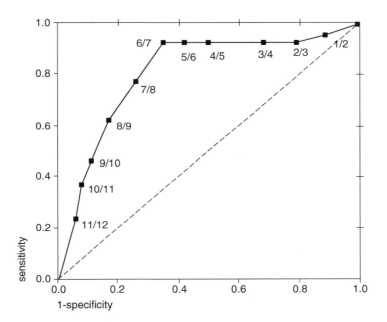

92. What is the above graph called?

A. Scatter plot
B. Funnel plot
C. Receiver operator characteristics curve
D. Galbraith plot
E. Forest plot

93. What does 1 – specificity represent?

A. False-positive rate
B. False-negative rate
C. True-positive rate
D. True-negative rate
E. None of the above

94. What does the dotted line represent?

 A. It is the curve of the test that best discriminates depressed from non-depressed people

 B. It is the curve of a test that partially discriminates depressed from non-depressed people

 C. It is the curve of a test that does not discriminate depressed from non-depressed people

 D. It is the curve representing the application of the current screening instrument to the whole population

 E. It is the curve of a test with maximum sensitivity but minimum specificity

95. Which cut-off point provides the best acceptable combination of sensitivity and specificity?

 A. 1/2

 B. 8/9

 C. 3/4

 D. 5/6

 E. 6/7

96. If the area under the curve (AUC) for the new test was found to be 0.5, what does it mean?

 A. The test can discriminate a depressed from a non-depressed person with high accuracy

 B. The test can discriminate a depressed from a non-depressed person with moderate accuracy

 C. The test cannot discriminate a depressed from a non-depressed person

 D. The test is half as good as the gold standard test

 E. The test can identify 50% of depressed patients correctly.

97–99 A meta-analysis of seven RCTs that compared a new antidepressant X with placebo was conducted. Effect size analysis for the change in HAMD scores are shown in the graph above. With respect to the graph below, answer Questions 97–99.

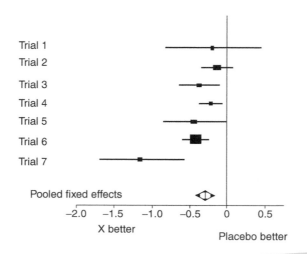

97. **What is the name of the graph shown above?**

    A. Funnel plot
    B. Galbraith plot
    C. L'Abbé plot
    D. Scatter plot
    E. Forest plot

98. **How many studies in the meta-analysis show statistically significant advantage for the new antidepressant?**

    A. 1
    B. 2
    C. 4
    D. 6
    E. 7

99. **Which of the trials has the greatest weight on the overall analysis?**

    A. Trial 1
    B. Trial 3
    C. Trial 4
    D. Trial 6
    E. Trial 7

100. **In which of the following situations is sensitivity analysis especially recommended while conducting a meta-analysis?**

    A. Presence of a high degree of homogeneity
    B. Any meta-analysis of continuous data
    C. Any meta-analysis of economic data
    D. Presence of significant publication bias
    E. Pooled outcome showing a large effect of intervention

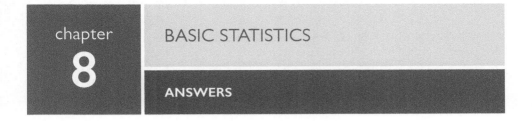

chapter

8

BASIC STATISTICS

ANSWERS

1. B. Internal validity is the degree to which a study establishes the cause-and-effect relationship between the treatment and the observed outcome. External validity is the degree to which the results of a study becomes applicable outside the experimental setting in which the study was conducted. In other words, external validity refers to generalizability of study results while internal validity refers to rigorousness of the research method. The benefit of agomelatine in different populations (choices A and E) refers to external validity; the cost of the drug and consistency of results obtained from different studies are related to applicability of the intervention in a clinical setting. Assessment of adherence to study protocol is one of many ways of analysing the quality of an intervention trial.

Slack MK and Drugalis JR. Establishing the internal and external validity of experimental studies. *American Journal of Health–Systems Pharm* 2001; **58**: 2173–2184.

2. C. Having a high positive predictive value, a likelihood ratio more than 10, and good inter-rater reliability as measured by kappa are desirable properties of an instrument. But when the same instrument is applied to a population with much lower prevalence of suicide (the studied phenomenon), the post-test probability decreases substantially. Post-test probability is a measure of positive predictive value in the target population; it depends on pretest probability, i.e. the prevalence and likelihood ratio.

Guyatt G and Rennie D, eds. *Users' Guides to the Medical Literature. A Manual for Evidence–Based Clinical Practice.* AMA Press, 2002, p. 130.

3. D. The likelihood ratio of a positive test (LR+) is the ratio between the probability of a positive test in a person with disease and the probability of a positive test in a person without disease. It can also be expressed as

LR+ = sensitivity/(1 − specificity)

Here, sensitivity = 0.8; specificity = 0.9.

Hence LR+ = 0.8/1 − 0.9 = 8.

Lawrie SM, McIntosh AM and Rao S. *Critical Appraisal for Psychiatry.* Churchill Livingstone, 2000. p. 97.

4. E. The NNT is the number of patients who will need the experimental treatment (X) for one additional patient to benefit compared with the control treatment. In the given trial, the response rate is characterized by a 50% drop in HAMD from baseline. Forty per cent of those taking drug X achieve this response. In contrast, this rate is 20% for the placebo. This means that 20% (40 – 20%) additional patients responded to the drug compared with placebo. In other words, if we treat another 100 patients with X, 20 extra patients will respond to X than those treated with a placebo. So we need to treat at least five people in order to see a benefit in one additional patient. This value five is known as the NNT. This can be calculated in another way. As you read further, you will note that 20% is the absolute benefit increase (ABI = EER – CER). And from the formula, NNT = 1/ABI, we get 1/20% = 5.

Cook RJ and Sackett DL. The number needed to treat: a clinically useful measure of treatment effect. *British Medical Journal* 1995; **310**: 452–454.

5. B. NNH is similar to the NNT. NNH is the number of patients who need to take the experimental treatment for one additional patient to experience an adverse effect. In the question, 20% of participants on X experienced suicidal ideas compared with 10% on placebo. Put in other words, the drug is responsible for suicidal ideas in an extra 10% of patients. So, if 100 patients receive the drug, 10 extra patients will experience suicidal ideas. That is, for every 10 people treated, one additional patient will experience suicidal ideas. Hence the NNH is 100/10 = 10. This obviously can be calculated from the formula NNH = 1/ARI (absolute risk increase) = 1/10% = 10. It is highly unlikely that X was marketed by the company.

Guyatt GH, Juniper EF, Walter SD, *et al*. Interpreting treatment effects in randomised trials. *British Medical Journal* 1998; **316**: 690–693.

6. C. This question tests one's ability to calculate post-test probability from likelihood ratios. The probability of having a disease after testing positive with a diagnostic test depends on two factors: (a) the prevalence of the disease, (b) the likelihood of a positive test result using the instrument. It is important to remember that baseline prevalence of a disease for which a diagnostic instrument is being tested is taken as the pretest probability.

So pretest probability = 10%

Now, post-test odds = likelihood ratio × pretest odds

From a given probability odds can be calculated using the formula

odds = (probability)/(1 – probability)

Here pretest odds = (10%)/(1 – 10%) = 10/90 = 1/9.

Now post-test odds = likelihood ratio × pretest odds

= 10 × 1/9 = 10/9

Using the formula probability = odds/(1 + odds)

post-test probability = (10/9)/[1 + (10/9)] = 10/19 = 52.3%

Guyatt G and Rennie D, eds. *Users' Guides to the Medical Literature. A Manual for Evidence-based Clinical Practice.* AMA Press, 2002, p. 660.

7. B. This question tests one's knowledge of the NNT (number needed to treat) concept. NNT is given by the inverse ratio of the absolute benefit increase (ABI) in therapeutic trials. ABI is the difference between benefit due to experimental intervention and the compared standard/placebo. Here it is given by 65% – 60% = 5%. If ABI = 5%, NNT = 100/5 = 20.

Guyatt G. and Rennie, D eds. *Users' Guides to the Medical Literature. A Manual for Evidence-based Clinical Practice.* AMA Press, 2002, p. 660.

8. C.   Threats to internal validity of an experimental study include confounding, selection bias, differential attrition, and quality of measurement. Having a significant difference in baseline SSRI therapy could explain differential outcomes in the trazodone vs temazepam groups. Similarly, poor randomization may lead to selection bias and influence the differences in outcome. Failure to account for differential drop-out rates may spuriously inflate or deflate the difference in outcome. Using a scale with poor sensitivity to change will reduce the magnitude of differences that could be observed. Given both groups are recruited from the same setting (hospital), this must not influence validity; on the other hand, this might well influence generalizability of results to the non-hospitalized population (external validity)

Campbell DT. Reforms as experiments. *American Psychologist* 1969; **24**: 409–429.
Slack MK and Draugalis JR. Establishing the internal and external validity of experimental studies. *American Journal of Health-System Pharmacy* 2001; **58**: 2173–2181.

9. A.   Published RCTs may quote impressive outcomes in terms of NNT. Applying principles of evidence-based medicine, one must check for the internal validity of a study and the degree of generalizability before adapting the results to clinical practice. One must also be aware of the fact that though clinically more meaningful, NNTs quoted in RCTs may not translate to the same extent in actual clinical practice. One way of appreciating the usefulness of a newly introduced drug is to calculate the NNT for one's own clinical population (target population). To enable this one may estimate the patient expected event rate (PEER), which is given by the expected spontaneous resolution rate or the response rate for an existing standard treatment. This can be obtained from the local audit data or clinical experience. The product of PEER and relative benefit increase from the published RCT gives the new absolute benefit increase (ABI new) value for the target population. The inverse of the new ABI gives the new NNT for the target population. The disease prevalence rate or absolute size of the target population has no effect on the new NNT.

Lawrie SM, McIntosh AM, Rao S. *Critical Appraisal for Psychiatry.* Churchill Livingstone, 2000, p. 117.

10. C.   In most treatment trials interventions are allocated by randomization. Block randomization and stratified randomization can be used to ensure the balance between groups in size and patient characteristics. But it is very difficult to stratify using several variables in a small sample. A widely acceptable alternative approach is minimization. This method can be used to ensure very good balance between groups for several confounding factors irrespective of the size of the sample. With minimization the treatment allocated to the next participant enrolled in the trial depends (wholly or partly) on the characteristics of those participants already enrolled. This is achieved by a simple mathematical computation of magnitude of imbalance during each allocation.

Altman DG. and Bland JM. Treatment allocation by minimisation. *British Medical Journal* 2005; **330**: 843.

11.A. RCTs provide high-quality evidence for or against proposed interventions. But RCTs have a major limitation in terms of generalizability. This is because the trials are conducted in a somewhat artificial experimental setting that is different from clinical practice. So RCTs have high internal validity due to rigorous methodology but poor external validity. Pragmatic RCTs are a type of RCTs introduced with the intention of increasing external validity, i.e. generalizability of RCT results. But this takes place at the expense of internal validity. In pragmatic RCTs the trial takes place in a setting as close as possible to natural clinical practice, i.e. the inclusion and exclusion criteria are less fastidious, often 'treatment as usual' is employed for comparisons, instead of placebos and real world, functionally significant outcomes are considered.

Hotopf M. The pragmatic randomised controlled trial. *Advances in Psychiatric Treatment* 2002; **8**: 326–333.

12. D. The power of a study refers to the ability of the study to show the difference in outcome between studied groups if such a difference actually exists. The term power calculation is often used while referring to sample size estimation before a study is undertaken. In order to carry out power calculation one has to know the expected precision and variance of measurements within the study sample (obtained from a literature search or pilot studies), the magnitude of a clinically significant difference, the certainty of avoiding type 1 error as reflected by the chosen p value, and the type of statistical test one will be performing. There is no point in calculating the statistical power once the results of a study are known. On completion of trials, measures such as confidence intervals indicate the power of a study and the precision of results.

Jones S, Carley S, and Harrison M. An introduction to power and sample size estimation. *Emergency Medicine Journal* 2003; **20**: 453–458.

13. E. Power refers to the probability of avoiding a type 2 error. To calculate power, one needs to know four variables.

1. sample size
2. magnitude of a clinically significant difference
3. probability of type 1 error (significance level from which p value is derived)
4. variance of the measure in the study sample.

Underpowered trials are those that enrol too few participants to identify differences between interventions (arbitrarily taken as at least 80% of the time) when such differences truly exist. Underpowered RCTs are prone to false-negative conclusions (type 2 errors). Somewhat controversially, underpowered trials are considered to be unethical, as they expose participants to the ordeals of research without providing an adequate contribution to clinical development.

Jones S, Carley S, and Harrison M. An introduction to power and sample size estimation. *Emergency Medicine Journal* 2003; **20**: 453–458.

14. D.   It is useful to construct a 2×2 table for calculating properties of reported diagnostic tests. From the given information we can draw the following:

	Schizophrenia	Controls	Total
Test positive	60	0	?
Test negative	?	?	?
Total	100	100	?

The remaining boxes can be filled as below

	Schizophrenia	Controls	Total
Test positive	60 (true positive)	0	60
Test negative	40	100 (true negative)	140
Total	100	100	200

Now, positive predictive value = true positive/total positive = 60/60 = 100%.

Guyatt G and Rennie D, eds. *Users' Guides to the Medical Literature. A Manual for Evidence-based Clinical Practice.* AMA Press, 2002, p. 661.

15. A.   Using the table from question 14

	Schizophrenia	Controls	Total
Test positive	60 (true positive)	0	60
Test negative	40	100 (true negative)	140
Total	100	100	200

Sensitivity = true positive/total diseased (schizophrenia subjects) = 60/100 = 60%

Guyatt G and Rennie D, eds. *Users' Guides to the Medical Literature. A Manual for Evidence-based Clinical Practice.* AMA Press, 2002, p. 661.

16. B.   Using the table from question 14,

	Schizophrenia	Controls	Total
Test positive	60 (true positive)	0 (false positive)	60
Test negative	40 (false negative)	100 (true negative)	140
Total	100	100	200

Accuracy = all true observations/total population studied = (100 + 60)/200 = 160/200 = 80%

Guyatt G and Rennie D, eds. *Users' Guides to the Medical Literature. A Manual for Evidence-based Clinical Practice.* AMA Press, 2002, p. 661.

17. D. This question asks the candidate to calculate the probability of a negative test in someone with the disorder – false-negative rate (FNR).

	Schizophrenia	Controls	Total
Test positive	60 (true positive)	0 (false positive)	60
Test negative	40 (false negative)	100 (true negative)	140
Total	100	100	200

This is given by FNR = false negative/total diseased = 40/100 = 40%

FNR is same as (1 – sensitivity); similarly false-positive rate (FPR) is same as (1 – specificity).

Guyatt G and Rennie D, eds. *Users' Guides to the Medical Literature. A Manual for Evidence-based Clinical Practice.* AMA Press, 2002, p. 661.

18. E. Sensitivity, specificity, and accuracy are measures that reflect the characteristics of the test instrument. These measures do not vary with changes in the disease prevalence. Positive predictive value increases while negative predictive value decreases with rising population prevalence of the disease studied. The prevalence can be interpreted as the probability before the test is carried out that the subject has the disease, known as the prior probability of disease. The positive and negative predictive values are the revised estimates of the same probability for those subjects who are positive and negative on the test, and are known as posterior probabilities. Thus the difference between the prior and posterior probabilities is one way of assessing the usefulness of the test.

Altman DG and Bland MJ. Statistics Notes: Diagnostic tests **2**: predictive values *British Medical Journal* 1994; **309**:102.

19. C. Agreement between different observers can be measured using the kappa (κ) statistic for categorical measures such as the one highlighted in this question (presence or absence of MRI hyperintensities). Kappa is a measure of the level of agreement in excess of that which would be expected by chance. It is calculated as the observed agreement in excess of chance, expressed as a proportion of the maximum possible agreement in excess of chance. In other words kappa = the difference between observed and expected agreement/(1 – expected agreement). In this example, the observed agreement is 78%. The expected agreement is 50%. Hence kappa = (0.78 – 0.50)/(1 – 0.50) = 0.28/0.50 = 56%.

Silman AJ and Macfarlane GJ. *Epidemiological studies: A Practical Guide,* 2nd edn. Cambridge University Press, 2004 p.125.

20. C. The median is calculated by placing observations in a rank order (either ascending or descending) and picking up the most central value. If the number of observations is even (multiples of two), then the median is taken as the arithmetic mean of the two middle values.

Lawrie SM, McIntosh AM, Rao S. *Critical Appraisal for Psychiatry.* Churchill Livingstone, 2000, p. 60.

21. A. The arithmetic mean is calculated from the sum of all individual observations divided by the number of observations. Here the number of observations = 5. The sum of individual observations = 12 + 12 + 14 + 16 + 21 = 75. The average = 75/5 = 15.

Lawrie SM, McIntosh AM, Rao S. *Critical Appraisal for Psychiatry.* Churchill Livingstone, 2000, p. 60.

22. B.   The probability that a test will provide a correct diagnosis is **not given** by the sensitivity or specificity of the test. Sensitivity and specificity are properties of the test instrument – they are not functions of the target population/clinical sample. On the other hand, positive and negative predictive values are functions of the population studied; they provide much more clinically useful information. Predictive values observed in one study do not apply universally. Positive predictive value increases with increasing prevalence of the disease; negative predictive value decreases with increasing prevalence. Sensitivity and specificity, being properties of the instrument used, do not vary with prevalence.

Altman DG and Bland JM. Diagnostic tests. 2. predictive values. *British Medical Journal* 1994; **309**: 102.

23. A.   The incremental cost-effectiveness ratio (ICER$_{AB}$) can be defined as the difference in cost (C) of interventions A and B divided by the difference in mean effectiveness (E), (C$_A$ – C$_B$)/ (E$_A$ – E$_B$), where intervention B is usually the placebo or standard intervention that is compared with intervention A. In this example, the difference in costs = \$680 – 400 = \$280. The difference in effectiveness as measured by percentage days of abstinence is 80 – 73% = 7%. Hence ICER = 280/7 = \$40 per patient per percentage point of days of abstinence.

Zarkin GA, Bray JW, Aldridge A, *et al.* Cost and cost-effectiveness of the COMBINE study in alcohol-dependent patients. *Archives of General Psychiatry* 2008; **65**: 1214–1221.

24. C.   When the relationship between two continuous variables is plotted in a graph, the resulting distribution may be a straight line or a curve. If the relationship between the independent (X) variable and dependent (Y) variable appear to follow a straight line, then linear regression can be constructed to predict the dependent variable from the independent variable. Otherwise, one can resort to one of the following methods:

1. Attempting to transform the available data to straighten the curved relationship.
2. One can try curvilinear regression, e.g. logarithmic regression, exponential regression, and trigonometric regression.
3. Unless there is a theoretical reason for supposing that a particular form of the equation as mentioned above, such as logarithmic or exponential, is needed, we usually test for non-linearity by using a polynomial regression equation.
4. Multiple linear regression is often used to examine the linear relationships when there is more than one independent variable influencing a dependent variable.

Bland M. *An Introduction to Medical Statistics*, 3rd edn. Oxford University Press, 2000, p. 314.

25. B.   The answer to this question can be found by calculating the number needed to treat (NNT). The absolute increase in benefit (ABI) is given by the difference in outcome between two groups. This is 20% as quoted by the drug representative. Hence NNT = 100/20 = 5. You need to treat five patients with the new drug to prevent one annual hospitalization. How small must the NNT be to be clinically impressive? This depends on the availability of other interventions and their NNTs, incremental cost of the proposed intervention, and tolerability of the intervention. The last one can be partly deciphered by calculating the number needed to harm for a notable side-effect of the intervention.

Guyatt G. and Rennie D, eds. *Users' Guides to the Medical Literature. A Manual for Evidence-based Clinical Practice.* AMA Press, 2002, p. 660.

26. D. Blinding reduces differential assessment of outcomes of interest (ascertainment bias, information bias, or observer bias) that can occur if the investigator or participant is aware of the group assignment. Blinding can also improve compliance and retention of trial participants and reduce unaccounted supplemental care or treatment that may be sought by the participants. Single blinding refers to either the investigator or the patient being blind to group assignment. Double blinding refers to both the patient and the investigator remaining unaware of the group assignment after randomization. This is desirable but not always possible in RCTs. In the example above, the subjects who undertake the exercise schedule cannot be kept unaware of exercising! A single-blind trial is possible in such cases.

Schulz KF and Grimes DA. Blinding in randomised trials: hiding who got what. *Lancet* 2002; **359**: 696–700.

27. C. MeSH stands for medical subject headings. It is a thesaurus embedded in the Pubmed–Medline interface and can be used to search literature more effectively using recognized key words.

Greenhalgh T. How to read a paper: the Medline database. *British Medical Journal* 1997; **315**: 180–183.

28. E. Single blind: either the patient or the clinician remains unaware of the intervention given.

Double blind: both the patient and investigator are unaware of the given intervention.

Open label: both researchers and the participants are aware of treatment being given after randomisation.

Triple blind: apart from the patient and the researcher, those who measure the study outcomes (the assessors) are also unaware of the given intervention.

Forder PM, Gebski VJ, and Keech AC. Allocation concealment and blinding: when ignorance is bliss. *Medical Journal of Australia* 2005; **182**: 87–89.

29. B. If random interchange between treatment and placebo groups occurs halfway through the study, this will lead to chaos and failed randomization. This is termed as contamination. This can occur when participants or their care givers discover they are 'controls', and obtain the experimental treatment outside the trial, thus effectively becoming the active treatment group. Choice C is practically impossible; to share controls of one RCT with another means the trial is open label. When each subject in the trial receives both intervention and placebo with a washout period in between while remaining blind to the intervention, this is called as crossover RCT. Crossover trials are possible only if short-term outcomes are evaluated in chronic diseases. This is because the disease process must be sufficiently long for the subject to receive both interventions across its course. Any intervention applied in a crossover setting must not permanently alter the disease process.

Sibbald B and Roberts C. Understanding controlled trials: Crossover trials. *British Medical Journal* 1998; **316**: 1719.

30. D. If one wishes to compare the effect of more than one intervention against placebo either a multi-arm RCT or a factorial design can be chosen. A multi-arm RCT is a simple extension of the usual RCTs where an extra arm of subjects is generated through randomization to allocate the second intervention in addition to placebo and the first intervention groups. A factorial RCT evaluates the effect of more than one intervention, independently and also in combination. In the above example the effect of two different psychotherapies independently and in combination could be studied using a factorial design.

Greenhalgh T. *How to Read a Paper: The Basics of Evidence Based Medicine*, 3rd edn. British Medical Journal, 2006, p. 45.

31. A. 'Degree of freedom' is defined as the number of values in the final calculation of statistics that are free to vary. In a two-way chi-square test, this is given by

Degrees of freedom (d.f.) = (number of rows − 1) × (number of columns − 1)

In this question, for a 2 × 2 table, there are 2 rows and 2 columns. Hence

d.f. = (2 − 1) × (2 − 1) = 1 × 1 = 1.

Degrees of freedom cannot take negative values.

Starr M and Chalmers I. The evolution of The Cochrane Library, 1988–2003. Update Software: Oxford (Accessed 6 September 2008 www.update–software.com/history/clibhist.htm).

32. B. No single study design is sufficient in itself to answer various clinical questions. For evaluation of a diagnostic test, a survey design that allows comparison with the gold standard is often used. For prognostic studies a prospective cohort design is useful. Therapeutic interventions are best evaluated using RCTs. Aetiological studies are often cohort or case–control studies; although the RCT is ideal it may not be always possible to conduct one. Epidemiological studies are often cross-sectional surveys.

Knottnerus JA and Muris JW (2003) Assessment of the accuracy of diagnostic tests: the cross-sectional study. *Journal of Clinical Epidemiology* **56**: 1118–1128.

33. D. The RCT has traditionally been considered as a study design that can yield results with a high degree of internal validity. But the major drawback of RCTs is that the process takes place under highly experimental conditions, which are not seen in clinical practice. So any results achieved from such RCTs, though valid, may not be reproducible in everyday practice. In order to circumvent this issue, more naturalistic trials that retain core principles of RCT such as randomization, longitudinal follow-up, and controlled intervention are being increasingly used. Such real-world RCTs are called pragmatic trials or effectiveness trials. Such trials can be useful to find out if an intervention will be *effective* in clinical practice, although they may not be suitable to study the biological *efficacy* of a drug. A pragmatic RCT may reject various practices seen in an explanatory RCT, such as strict exclusion criteria, blinding, placebo use, fixed dose intervention, high follow-up care, per-protocol analysis, etc. But basic principles such as randomization and use of probability theory (hypothesis testing and p values) are retained.

Hotopf M. The pragmatic randomised controlled trial. *Advances in Psychiatric Treatment* 2002; **8**: 326–333.

34. C. Bias is defined as any trend in the collection, analysis, interpretation, publication, or review of data that can lead to conclusions that are systematically different from the truth. It can also be termed as a systematic error that influences the result in either direction. Hence a biased study could either overestimate or underestimate the true effect, depending on the direction of the trend. Bias may be introduced by poor study design or poor data collection. Bias cannot be 'controlled for' at the analysis stage. In RCTs, randomization ensures a reduction in selection bias if the process is carried out in a strictly concealed manner. Blinding can reduce the measurement bias if properly executed.

Page LA and Henderson M. Appraising the evidence: what is measurement bias? *Evidence Based Mental Health* 2008; **11**: 36–37.

35. E. Recall bias refers to the systematic error produced by the tendency of subjects to recall an exposure differently when they are diseased compared with when they are not. Recall bias most often occurs in case–control studies. The remaining choices refer to genuine disadvantages of a well-conducted RCT.

Lawrie SM, McIntosh AM and Rao S. *Critical Appraisal for Psychiatry*. Churchill Livingstone, 2000, p. 47.

36. D.   In most drug trials, patients drop-out because of non-efficacy or adverse events. If we think that a number of participants drop-out because of non-efficacy, dropping them out of the analysis would project a favourable outcome for the drug in question. Hence the LOCF method takes the last observation and utilizes it in the analysis. For illustration, we take two subjects, in a trial of antidepressants.

Antidepressant trial Montgomery–Asberg depression rating scale (MADRS)

	Subject 1	Subject 2
Baseline	30	30
Week 1	20	30
Week 2	10	30 (drop-out due to non efficacy)
Week 3	5	30
Final score	1	30

Subject 1, improves significantly over the 4 weeks, his MADRS score has dropped to 1 from a baseline of 30, while Subject 2 dropped out of the study in the second week, due to non-efficacy. If we remove subject 2 from the analysis, the mean score at the end would be 1 (an whopping improvement of 29 points on the MADRS), while if we carry forward his last observation score (week 2) of 30 to the end and took the mean of the two scores (15.05), the drop is only 15 points from the mean baseline score of 30.

Trials of Alzheimer's disease interventions are different, since we do not expect (although we most definitely would like to see) improvement in the cognitive score, but a rather slow decline in scores over time, in spite of the medications, due to the progressive nature of the illness. If a patient drops out early because of the experience of adverse effects, carrying forward his score to the endpoint analysis will falsely project a favourable outcome. Again to illustrate, let us consider a trial of cholinesterase inhibitors.

ChI trial MMSE

	Subject 1	Subject 2
Baseline	20	20
Week 1	20	20 (drops out because of side effects)
Week 2	10	20
Week 3	5	20
Final score	1	20

Subject 1 experienced a decline of 19 points over 4 weeks, while the second subject dropped out the first week, when his MMSE had not declined. If we carry forward his last observation of 20, it will look like there was no deterioration at all, and the difference in the mean scores over time would be diluted to 10, rather than a drop of 19.

As a corollary, the reason for drop-out is another important issue. In trials of Alzheimer's disease interventions, early drop-outs are most probably due to adverse effects, while late drop-outs are due to non-efficacy. This can again project a favourable outcome for the drug.

Streiner DL. The case of the missing data: methods of dealing with dropouts and other research vagaries. Can J Psychiatry 2002; **47**:68–75.

37. E. There are a number of ways to manage heterogeneity. The easiest way would be to avoid it. This includes using strict inclusion criteria to include studies that are as similar as possible. In case of continuous variables, one of the ways would be to transform the data so that all data look similar and are less heterogeneous. Meta regression is a collection of statistical procedures to assess heterogeneity, in which the effect size of study is regressed on one or several covariates, with a value defined for each study. The fixed-effect model of meta-analysis as reported in this question, considers the variability between the studies as exclusively due to random variation. The random-effects model assumes a different underlying effect for each study and takes this into consideration as an additional source of variation. The effects of the studies are assumed to be randomly distributed and the central point of this distribution is the focus of the combined (pooled) effect estimate. If there were some types of studies that were likely to be quite different from the others, a subgroup analysis may be done. And finally, one could exclude the studies that contribute a great deal to the heterogeneity. Locating unpublished studies may help reduce publication bias but will not have any predictable and constant effect on the degree of heterogeneity.

Freemantle N and Geddes J. Understanding and interpreting systematic reviews and meta–analyses. Part 2. Meta-analyses (editorial). *Evidence-Based Mental Health* 1998; **1**: 102–4.

Geddes J, Freemantle N, Streiner D, *et al*. Understanding and interpreting systematic reviews and meta–analyses. Part 1. Rationale, search strategy, and describing results (editorial). *Evidence-Based Mental Health* 1998; **1**: 68–9.

38. C. Odds are the probability of an event occurring divided by the probability of the event not occurring. An odds ratio is the odds of the event in one group (e.g. intervention group) divided by the odds in another group (e.g. control group). Odds ratios tend to exaggerate the true relative risk to some degree. But this exaggeration is kept minimal and even negligible if the probability of the studied outcome is low (empirically, less than 10%); in such cases the odds ratio approximates the true relative risk. As the event becomes more common the odds ratio no longer remains a useful proxy for the relative risk. It is suggested that the use of odds ratios should probably be limited to case-control studies and logistic regression examining dichotomous variables. As risk refers to the probability of an event occurring at a time point, in other words it is the same as the incidence rate. The inherent cross-sectional nature of a case–control study (where 'existing cases' are recruited) does not allow one to study 'new' incidences. Hence we cannot measure risk, and so relative risk, from case–control designs.

Katz KA. The (relative) risks of using odds ratios. *Archives of Dermatology* 2006; **142**: 761–764.

39. E. Choice A refers to a clinical question related to therapeutic intervention – RCTs are best suited to answer this. Choice B is an epidemiological question – 'how many in a population have a particular condition?' A cross-sectional survey could answer this question. Choice C refers to a prognostic question – how long will it take for schizoaffective relapse following lithium discontinuation? A prospective cohort (or a RCT if ethically approved) is the most appropriate design for this question. Choice D requires a clinical audit, which is often closer to a cross-sectional survey in design. Choice E refers to defined cases and controls being compared for a possible exposure or risk factor that might have occurred in the past. Hence the case–control design is best suited to answer this question. Please note that it is possible to design a prospective cohort study by observing for a long time those with academic failure to detect development of depression.

Lawrie SM and McIntosh AM, Rao S. *Critical Appraisal for Psychiatry*. Churchill Livingstone, 2000, p. 27.

40. B.   N-of-1 trials are randomized double-blind multiple crossover comparisons of an active drug against placebo in a single patient. The design uses a series of pairs of treatment periods called modules. Within each module the patient receives active treatment during one period and either an accepted standard treatment or placebo in the other. Random allocation determines the order of the two treatment periods within each pair and both clinician and patient are blinded for the intervention. This design is mostly suited for chronic recurrent conditions for which long-term interventions exist that are not curative. Interventions with rapid onset and offset of effects are best suited for n-of-1 trials. This allows shorter treatment periods wherein multiple modules of intervention and placebo/standard treatment can be compared, increasing the chance of achieving a statistically significant result. It is also necessary that the interventions tested must be cleared from the patient's system within a finite washout period.

Price JD and Evans JG. An N-of-1 randomized controlled trial ('N-of-1 trial') of donepezil in the treatment of non–progressive amnestic syndrome. *Age and Ageing* 2002; **31**: 307–309.

41. E.   Publication bias refers to the tendency of journals to accept and publish certain types of studies more often than the others. In general, studies with results that are impressively significant or of higher quality by virtue of larger sample size are more successful in getting published. Publication bias can be considered as a form of selection bias when one attempts a systematic review or meta-analysis. Publication bias can be detected using a funnel plot – visual inspection of a graph drawn by plotting a measure of precision (often sample size) against treatment effect will reveal asymmetry of the two arms of the funnel-shaped graph if publication bias is present. Galbraith plot refers to a graph obtained by plotting a measure of precision such as (1/standard error) against standard normal deviate (log of odds ratio/standard error). The coordinates obtained from such a plot can be used to determine the extent of publication bias using linear regression. Failsafe N is another way of estimating publication bias. Consider a meta-analysis yielding a statistically significant difference in outcome between two interventions, despite suspected publication bias. Then failsafe N answers the question 'How many missing studies are needed to reduce the effect to statistical non-significance?' The higher the failsafe N, the lower the publication bias. If one could solicit and compare all unpublished data with published data, then publication bias would become obvious.

Lawrie SM, McIntosh AM, and Rao S. *Critical Appraisal for Psychiatry*. Churchill Livingstone, 2000, p. 146.

42. A.   Allocation concealment refers to the process used to prevent fore knowledge of the assignment before allocation is complete. So the investigator who recruits subjects for a trial will not know the nature of assignment of consequent subjects that enter randomization. Allocation concealment seeks to prevent selection bias, protects the allocation sequence *before and until* assignment, and can almost *always* be successfully implemented in a RCT. It is often confused with blinding which seeks to prevent ascertainment bias and protects the sequence *after* allocation, and cannot always be implemented.

Schulz KF, Chalmers I., and Altman DG. The landscape and lexicon of blinding in randomized trials. *Annals of Internal Medicine* 2002; **136**: 254–259.

43. B.   The standard deviation has the same units as the primary variable. This is an advantage of standard deviation compared with variance, which is also a measure of dispersion.

Lawrie SM, McIntosh AM, and Rao S. *Critical Appraisal for Psychiatry*. Churchill Livingstone, 2000, p. 60.

44. D. If many observations are substantially higher than the median we can assume that the mean of the distribution might be greater than the median. This translates to a positively skewed distribution. No comments can be made on mode using the available information.

Lawrie SM, McIntosh AM, and Rao S. *Critical Appraisal for Psychiatry.* Churchill Livingstone, 2000, p. 60.

45. C. α is the probability of type 1 error. It is used to set the threshold for statistical (not clinical) significance, often arbitrarily set as p = 0.01–0.05 (α = 1–5%). If α = 0.05, there is a 1 in 20 or 5% chance that the null hypothesis is rejected wrongly.

Lawrie SM, McIntosh AM, and Rao S. *Critical Appraisal for Psychiatry.* Churchill Livingstone, 2000, p. 64.

46. C. Despite the increasing importance and abundance of systematic reviews and meta-analyses in the scientific literature, the reporting quality of systematic reviews varies widely. To address the issue of suboptimal reporting of meta-analyses, an international group in 1996 developed a guidance called the QUOROM Statement (**QU**ality **O**f **R**eporting **O**f **M**eta-analyses). QUOROM focused on the standards of reporting meta-analyses of RCTs. A revision of these guidelines renamed as PRISMA (Preferred Reporting Items for Systematic reviews and Meta-Analyses) includes several conceptual advances in the methodology of systematic reviews.

Moher D, Cook DJ, Eastwood S, *et al.* Improving the quality of reporting of meta–analysis of randomized controlled trials: The QUOROM statement. *Lancet* 1994; **354**: 1896–1900.
David Moher *et al.*, 'Preferred Reporting Items for Systematic Reviews and Meta–Analyses: The PRISMA Statement,' *PLoS Med* **6**: e1000097.

47. E. Meta-analysis is generally done to combine the results of different trials, as individual clinical trials are often too small and hence underpowered to detect treatment effects reliably. Meta-analysis increases the power of statistical analyses by pooling the results of all available trials. But this comes at a small cost. Although similar studies are taken to be included in the meta-analysis, it is likely that each trial is different from each other just by chance. Sometimes the difference can occur due to foreseeable situations, e.g. the dosage of medication tested, the mean ages of the population tested, difference in the scales used, etc, may differ among studies. To measure if this heterogeneity is more than the random heterogeneity we expect, statisticians resort to certain tests of heterogeneity. They are statistical as in the chi-square test (or Q statistic), which tests the 'null hypothesis" of homogeneity and the I-squared test (which measures the amount of variability due to heterogeneity). Galbraith's plot and l'Abbé plot are pictorial representations of heterogeneity. A paired t test is generally not used to calculate the heterogeneity.

Perera R, and Heneghan C. Interpreting meta-analysis in systematic reviews. *Evidence-Based Medicine* 2008; **13**: 67–69.
Lam RW. Using metaanalysis to evaluate evidence: practical tips and traps. *Canadian Journal of Psychiatry* **50**: 167–174.

48. A. Data can be qualitative or quantitative. Quantitative data refers to measures that often have a meaningful unit of expression. This can be either discrete or continuous. A discrete measure has no other observable value between two contiguous potentially observable values, i.e. there are 'gaps' between values. A continuous variable, on the other hand, can take potentially infinite values. The other choices in the question refer to qualitative measures whose value can only be described and counted but cannot be expressed in meaningful units.

Lawrie SM, McIntosh AM and Rao S. *Critical Appraisal for Psychiatry.* Churchill Livingstone, 2000, p. 56.

49. A.   A major disadvantage with RCTs is the poor generalizability of experimental findings to a clinical setting. Having strict inclusion and exclusion criteria may help chose a highly homogeneous population, increasing the internal validity of the study but at the expense of generalizability.

Persaud, N. and Mamdani, M.M. External validity: the neglected dimension in evidence ranking. Journal of Evaluation in Clinical Practice 2006:12(4); 450– 453.

50. C.   In scientific research, nothing can be proven; we can only disprove presumed facts. If one wants to prove maternal smoking causes school refusal, it is best to assume that maternal smoking does not cause school refusal to start with and then proceed to disprove this statement. Such statements waiting to be disproved during the course of a research study are called the null hypotheses. The converse of the null hypothesis is called the alternative hypothesis.

Research question: Does maternal smoking increase risk of school refusal?

Null hypothesis: Maternal smoking does not increase risk of school refusal

Alternative hypothesis: Maternal smoking increases the risk of school refusal.

Guyatt G and Rennie D, eds. *Users' Guides to the Medical Literature. A Manual for Evidence-based Clinical Practice.* AMA Press, 2002, p. 680.

51. D.   Subjects do not get randomized in a simple cohort study. Hence there is no question of allocation concealment. When valid instruments and a reasonable follow-up schedule are used, identification of those who develop the 'event' of interest/outcome is often not difficult in a cohort design. Often the most difficult part is to identify a reasonable control cohort that lacks the 'exposure' of interest. Internal controls refer to those who are 'non-exposed' but derived from the same study population as the 'exposed'. External control refers to an independently recruited cohort without the exposure.

Lawrie SM, McIntosh AM, and Rao S. *Critical Appraisal for Psychiatry.* Churchill Livingstone, 2000, p. 29.

52. D.   95% confidence limits of means of a sample are nothing but the range between an observation less than approximately two standard error units less than mean value and an observation two standard error units more than the mean value. Using mathematical expression, 95% confidence limits = mean ± (2 × standard error of mean).

Standard error of mean is calculated as SE = standard deviation/√sample size.

SE = 15/√36 = 15/6 = 2.5 in this question.

Hence 95% confidence limits are

262 ± (2 × 2.5) = 262 ± 5 = 257, 267.

Bland, M. An Introduction to Medical Statistics, 3rd edn. Oxford University Press, 2000. P. 126.

53. B.   An important property of the normal distribution curve is the relationship between the SD of normally distributed observations and probability. Normal distribution curves are symmetric and bell-shaped. Nearly 68.5% of the sampled population will lie within 1 SD of the mean on either side of the curve, 95.5% within 2 SDs, and 99% within 3 SDs. In other words, there is a 1% chance that an observation will fall outside +3 SD to −3 SD; a 5% chance that it will fall outside +2SD to −2SD and nearly 30% chance that it will occur outside +1SD and −1SD.

Johnstone EC, et al., eds. *Companion to Psychiatric Studies*, 7th edn. Churchill Livingstone, 2004, p. 189.

54. C. If the confidence interval includes a null treatment effect, the null hypothesis cannot be rejected within the set levels of confidence limits. Confidence intervals provide a measure of dispersion of the point estimate within stipulated confidence limits (arbitrarily 95% corresponds to a p value of 5%). In other words, confidence intervals provide the assured range within which the true value may lie. Confidence intervals are a measure of precision of the results obtained from a study. The larger the sample studied, the narrower the intervals. If the confidence intervals cross the value '0' for the difference between means then the results are statistically not significant. If it crosses the value '1' for ratio measures such as the odds ratio, it is not significant. If it crosses infinity for inverse ratios such as NNT then it is not significant.

Johnstone EC, et al., eds. *Companion to Psychiatric Studies*, 7th edn. Churchill Livingstone, 2004, p. 192.

55. A. In this study, the dependent variable is treated as a categorical outcome. In other words, the population has been categorized into 'akathisia present' or 'akathisia absent'. This type of outcome yields frequency counts or proportions that can be analysed for significance using the chi square test. The t test is used for comparing means. The Wilcoxon rank sum test is a non-parametric equivalent of the t test. Pearson coefficients are used to analyse correlation. Regression analyses are used to predict one variable from another when they are correlated.

Johnstone EC, et al., eds. *Companion to Psychiatric Studies*, 7th edn. Churchill Livingstone, 2004, p. 193.

56. D. Irrespective of the number of observations made, the shape of a normally distributed curve is symmetric and bell shaped. The exact shape of the normal distribution is defined by a function that has only two parameters: mean and standard deviation. For a given range of scores, when the standard deviation is small, the curve becomes leptokurtic, i.e. thin but still symmetric. When the standard deviation is larger, it becomes platykurtic.

Lawrie SM, McIntosh AM, and Rao S. *Critical Appraisal for Psychiatry*. Churchill Livingstone, 2000, p. 255.

57. C. Standard deviation is a widely used measure of dispersion of data in *descriptive statistics*. Other measures include range, interquartile range (usually accompanies median values), and variance. Standard deviation is obtained by the root mean square of differences between individual observations and the mean value. Note that standard error is often preferred as the measure of dispersion while making inferences from a sample of the population. Standard error is a measure of precision of sample estimate in comparison with the population value.

Johnstone EC, et al., eds. *Companion to Psychiatric Studies*, 7th edn. Churchill Livingstone, 2004, p. 190.

58. B. The iterative approach in qualitative studies refers to the process of altering the research methods and building the hypothesis as the study progresses, in response to new information gained while conducting the research. This flexibility allows qualitative studies to follow an inductive rather than the deductive approach seen in quantitative research. Data come before theory is generated in inductive methods; a stated theory is tested using generated data in deductive methods.

Greenhalgh T. How to read a paper: papers that go beyond numbers. *British Medical Journal* 1997; **315**: 740–743.

59. E. In the above question, the mean is given as 120 mmHg. Assuming normal distribution with a standard deviation of 10 mmHg, we can find out the proportion of the population that will fall between two observed values. For values between −1 and +1 standard deviation from the mean, this will be nearly 68%. Nearly 34% will have values between the mean and 1 standard deviation. In other words 34% will have systolic blood pressure between 120 mmHg and 130 mmHg.

Lawrie SM, McIntosh AM, and Rao S. *Critical Appraisal for Psychiatry.* Churchill Livingstone, 2000, p. 60.

60. A. Significant numbers of subjects recruited for trials often do not complete the trial as per protocol. The data generated from such drop-outs cannot be ignored as this will potentially lead to an attrition bias in favour of the intervention generally. Therefore, it is a standard practice to analyse the results of trials on an 'intention to treat' basis, i.e. data from subjects are analysed as per initial allocation irrespective of trial completion. In a few situations such as the 'efficacy studies', intention to treat analysis is not used, instead 'per-protocol analysis' is carried out.
An efficacy study is designed to explain the effects of the intervention itself. This is in contrast to effectiveness studies, which are designed to study the usefulness of making an intervention available (choices B, C and D).

Greenhalgh T. Assessing the methodological quality of published papers. *British Medical Journal* 1997;**315**:305–8.

61. D. Relative risk reduction (or relative benefit increase) is calculated using the following expression: relative risk reduction = absolute risk reduction/control event rate (RRR = ARR/CER)

The control event rate is 20%; the experimental event rate is 40%.

Absolute risk reduction is the difference between the two event rates, i.e. 40 − 20 = 20%
RRR = 20/20 = 1

Guyatt G and Rennie D, eds. *Users' Guides to the Medical Literature. A Manual for Evidence-based Clinical Practice.* AMA Press, 2002, p. 660.

62. B. The NNT can be calculated from the absolute risk reduction (ARR).
NNT = 1/ARR
NNT = 1/0.2 = 5

Five subjects must be treated with memantine to have one additional response.

Guyatt G and Rennie D, eds. *Users' Guides to the Medical Literature. A Manual for Evidence-based Clinical Practice.* AMA Press, 2002, p. 660.

63. A. To calculate the odds ratio, it will be useful to construct a 2 × 2 table. As per protocol analysis is used, only those who completed the trial have been included in the analysis.

	Response	No response	Total
Memantine	40 (a)	60 (b)	100
Placebo	20 (c)	80 (d)	100
Total			

The odds ratio is obtained using the cross product ratio ad/bc
= (80 × 40)/(60 × 20) = 8/3 = 2.7

Guyatt G and Rennie D, eds. *Users' Guides to the Medical Literature. A Manual for Evidence-based Clinical Practice.* AMA Press, 2002, p. 660.

64. C.   Spearman's correlation is used for non-parametric correlation analysis. It is also called the rank correlation test. It can be used when one or both variables to be correlated consist of ranks (ordinal) or if they exist as quantitative data but do not have normal distribution. Pearson's correlation is used for parametric correlation. Kappa is a measure of agreement not correlation. Cohen's d is used to calculate effect size. The internal consistency of an instrument is tested using Cronbach's alpha.

Lawrie SM, McIntosh AM, and Rao S. *Critical Appraisal for Psychiatry*. Churchill Livingstone, 2000, pp. 72 and 75.

65. B.   To enable use of inferential statistics, standard sampling assumptions such as (1) the randomness of the sampled data and (2) the independent nature of the observations must be met. In addition, when parametric statistics are employed assumptions such as

1. homogeneity of variance of the samples
2. observations are obtained from continuous (interval/ratio) scales
3. normal distribution of the observed variable

must be met. There is no set proportion of population size that must constitute the sample size in order to use parametric statistics. But in samples that are too small the distribution may not be normal and the central limit theorem may not be applicable. In conditions where such assumptions are not met non-parametric statistics are used. The latter are often considered to be less robust.

Bland, M. *An Introduction to Medical Statistics*, 3rd edn. Oxford University Press, 2000, p. 210.

66. A.   Drawing a 2 × 2 table will help answering this question

	Death	No death	Total
Drug A	20		200
Placebo	25		225
Total			

Further information can be filled in as below:

	Death	No death	Total
Drug A	20	180	200
Placebo	25	200	225
Total	45	380	425

Control event rate is the rate of death ('event' of interest) in the control group = 25/225

Guyatt G and Rennie D, eds. *Users' Guides to the Medical Literature. A Manual for Evidence-based Clinical Practice*. AMA Press, 2002, p. 660.

67. C.   Adequacy of blinding can be tested during or after completing a trial by asking the blinded parties to guess the allocation. Guess rates that are significantly higher than expected by chance indicate failure of blinding. Testing for 'blindness' may not generate valid answers all the time. This is because as participants begin to experience treatment response or outcomes of interest, they begin to generate 'hunches' about the efficacy of the treatments being tested. Hence tests for blinding can show spurious failure of blinding while in fact they test the 'efficacy hunches' that develop late in the process of a trial.

Sackett DL. Measuring the success of blinding in RCTs: don't, must, can't or needn't? *International Journal of Epidemiology* 2007; **36**: 664–665.

68. B. The central limit theorem explains why normal distributions are so frequent when considering most biological parameters. Consider repeated sampling from a population where distribution of the observed variable is unknown. You intend to plot the distribution of individual means of each sample from the population. As sample size increases, the sample means approach a normal distribution with its mean value being the same as the population mean and a standard deviation equal to the standard deviation of the population divided by the square root of the sample size. Usually 10 or more observations are sufficient to result in an approximate normal distribution.

Lawrie SM, McIntosh AM, and Rao S. *Critical Appraisal for Psychiatry*. Churchill Livingstone, 2000, p. 252.

69. C. The term validity refers to the strength of our conclusions, or in the case of statistics, the strength of our inferences. It refers to applicability. The term reliability refers to the consistency of our measurements, or the reproducibility. An important subtype of validity is called criterion validity. If an instrument provides a result that withstands the test of an external criterion then the instrument is said to have high criterion validity. The external criterion may be a measurement that can be obtained more or less at the same time (concurrent validity) or it may be an outcome that is predicted to occur in the future (predictive validity). If a test offers something over and above what is offered by an existing instrument, then incremental validity can be established. Internal consistency of a test refers to looking at how consistent the results are for different items (measuring the same construct) within the instrument studied. This can be measured by undertaking item–item correlation, item–total score correlation or split half reliability (Cronbach's alpha; see elsewhere in this chapter).

Fitzner K. Reliability and validity: a quick review. *Diabetes Educator* 2007; **33**: 775–780.

70. E. Questions similar to this are very common in the MRCPsych exam. Most of such questions provide some data and require the candidate to do a series of calculations from the data. It is always advisable to redraw as soon as possible the presented data in a format that will fit the purpose. From the given table we can create a 2×2 table, with the gold standard result on the top. One should be careful while constructing the 2×2 table. It is advisable to stick to one style of using columns and rows to indicate a particular group of data. Here, we have drawn the 2×2 table with the gold standard results indicated across the two data columns with screening test results indicated across the two rows.

		DSM-IV (gold standard)		
		Diagnosis present	Diagnosis absent	Total
Screening test	Positive	(A) 39	(B) 40	(A+B) 79
	Negative	(C) 4	(D) 84	(C+D) 88
	Total	(A+C) 43	(B+D) 124	167

Sensitivity is defined as the test's ability to identify people who, according to the *diagnostic (gold) standard*, actually have the disorder (true positives). Sensitivity = A/(A + C) = 39/43 = 90.69%, i.e. 90.69% of subjects who really have depression according to DSM-IV criteria have a positive test result on the screening test. In other words, sensitivity is the proportion of true positives (cases) correctly identified by the test.

Streiner D and Geddes J. Some useful concepts and terms used in articles about diagnosis. *Evidence-Based Mental Health* 1998; **1**: 6–8.

71. A. Specificity is defined as the test's ability to exclude people who, according to the diagnostic (gold) standard, do not actually have the disorder (true negatives). Specificity = D/(B + D) = 84/124 = 67.74%, i.e. 67.74% of the people who do not have depression will have a negative result on the two-question screen. Thus specificity is the proportion of true negatives among all non-diseased individuals. In other words, it is the ability of a test to rule out the disorder among people who do not have it.

Streiner D and Geddes J. Some useful concepts and terms used in articles about diagnosis. *Evidence-Based Mental Health* 1998; **1**: 6–8.

72. A.　Not all of those people, who have been found to be 'positive' on the test, might *actually have* the disorder. Positive predictive value (PPV) gives the proportion of true positives among the test positives. It is calculated using the formula, PPV = A/(A + B) = 39/79 = 49.36%, i.e. 49.36% of people diagnosed with depression using the screening test actually have the illness.

Streiner D and Geddes J. Some useful concepts and terms used in articles about diagnosis. *Evidence-Based Mental Health 1998*; **1**: 6–8.

73. E.　Not all of the people who have been found to be 'negative' on the test might *actually be disease free*. Negative predictive value (NPV) answers the question 'Of those people who have been found to be 'disease negative' on the test, how many *actually do not have* the disorder?' It is calculated using the formula, NPV = D/(C + D) = 84/88 = 95.45%, i.e. 95.45% of people diagnosed 'normal' on the test don't have the disorder.

Streiner D and Geddes J. Some useful concepts and terms used in articles about diagnosis. *Evidence-Based Mental Health* 1998; **1**: 6–8.

74. D.　The prevalence, also known as the pretest probability or base rate, refers to the proportion of people who have the disorder = (A + C)/N, i.e. 43/167 = 25.74%.

Streiner D and Geddes J. Some useful concepts and terms used in articles about diagnosis. *Evidence-Based Mental Health* 1998; **1**: 6–8.

75. A.　PPV and NPV depend on the prevalence of the illness, and, as one can see, the prevalence of an illness can vary according to the population it tests. For example, the prevalence of depression is likely to be more in patients in a palliative care unit. Since the prevalence keeps changing with population, and hence the PPV and NPV, one way of summarizing the findings of a study of a diagnostic test where there is a different prevalence is to use the *likelihood ratio*. The *likelihood ratio for a positive test (LR+) result* is the likelihood that a positive test comes from a person with the disorder rather than one without the disorder. LR+ is calculated using the formula, LR+ve = [A/(A + C)]/[B/(B + D)]

or simply

LR+ve = sensitivity/(1 - specificity).

So, (39/43)/(40/124) = 0.90/0.322 = 2.8. Since the specificity and sensitivity of a test are considered to be constant for any particular test, the LR is also constant irrespective of prevalence rates.

Streiner D and Geddes J. Some useful concepts and terms used in articles about diagnosis. *Evidence-Based Mental Health*1998; **1**: 6–8.

76. A.   The LR– represents the likelihood that a *negative test* comes from a person *with the disorder* rather than one without the disorder. LR– is calculated using the formula LR–ve = [C/(A + C)]/[D/(B + D)], or simply LR–ve = (1 – sensitivity)/specificity.

So, (4/43)/(84/124) = 0.10/0.67 = 0.14

Similar to LR+ve, LR–ve is also constant irrespective of prevalence rates.

Streiner D and Geddes J. Some useful concepts and terms used in articles about diagnosis. *Evidence-Based Mental Health* 1998; **1**: 6–8.

77. E.   The post-test probability is the probability that a patient, scoring positive on the test, actually has the disorder (PPV). It can be calculated using the nomogram that is provided. Since we know the pre-test probability (prevalence) and the likelihood ratio, we should be able to find the post-test probability from the chart. A straight line drawn through the pre-test probability (25) and the likelihood ratio +ve (2.8) should yield a post-test probability of about 50.

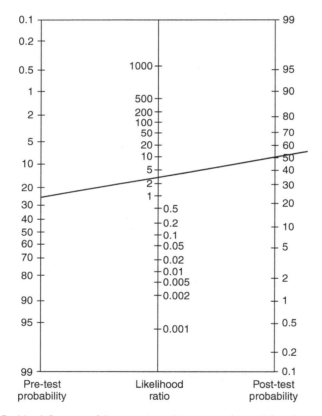

Streiner D and Geddes J. Some useful concepts and terms used in articles about diagnosis. *Evidence-Based Mental Health* 1998; **1**: 6–8.
Fagan TJ. *New England Journal of Medicine* 1975; **293**: 257.

78. B. In this case, since the question is about post-test probability of a negative test, the likelihood ratio −ve (0.14) and the line would pass through 4.

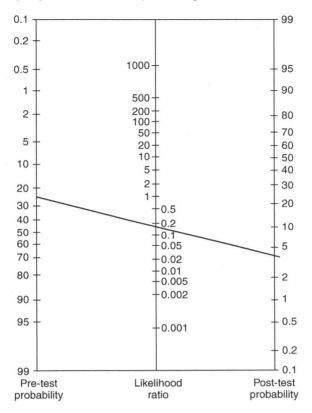

Streiner D and Geddes J. Some useful concepts and terms used in articles about diagnosis. *Evidence-Based Mental Health* 1998; **1**: 6–8.

79. A. False positive (FP) is the number of people diagnosed to have a condition with the new test when they actually do not have the condition according to the gold standard. In this case, the percentage of people falsely identified by the test as depressed. Using the 2 × 2 table, false positive is calculated FP = B/B+D = 40/124 = 32%.

Streiner D and Geddes J. Some useful concepts and terms used in articles about diagnosis. *Evidence-Based Mental Health* 1998; **1**: 6–8.

80. B. False negative (FN) is the number of people not diagnosed with a condition with the new test when they actually have the condition according to the gold standard. In this case, the percentage of people among the depressed group falsely identified by the test as not depressed, i.e. C/A +C; 4/43 = 9.3%.

Streiner D and Geddes J. Some useful concepts and terms used in articles about diagnosis. *Evidence-Based Mental Health* 1998; **1**: 6–8.

81. D. In Question 75, we discussed how the prevalence of a condition can vary according to the population tested. Using the same screening test for depression in the general population of 1000 subjects (N), we are asked to calculate the positive predictive value. The prevalence rate or pre-test probability is 10% (A + C/N). We need to make a fresh 2 × 2 table in order to answer the question. We know that sensitivity and specificity remains constant for the disease. From the given data the prevalence = A+C/N = 10%

As N = 1000 now, we can say A+C = 100

Sensitivity (A/A+C) = A/100 = 0.91; so, A = 91.

Specificity (D/B+D) = 67.74%; D/900 = 0.677; D = 610.

		DSM-IV (gold standard)		
		Diagnosis present	Diagnosis absent	Total
Screening Test	Positive	(A) 91	(B) 290	(A+B) 381
	Negative	(C) 9	(D) 610	(C+D) 619
	Total	(A+C) 100	(B+D) 900	1000

Using the formula for positive predictive value, PPV = A/A+B = 91/290 = 31%.

Streiner D and Geddes J. Some useful concepts and terms used in articles about diagnosis. *Evidence-Based Mental Health* 1998; **1**: 6–8.

82. E. See the table in Answer 81. Using the formula for negative predictive value, NPV = D/C+D = 98.36%. Note that the same answer can be derived using pretest odds and likelihood ratios. Please see question 6.

Streiner D and Geddes J. Some useful concepts and terms used in articles about diagnosis. Evidence-Based Mental Health 1998; **1**:6–8.

83. A. This question pertains to the risk of the development of dyspepsia in the trial.
As mentioned earlier, a 2 × 2 table with the exposure (drug/placebo) to the left and the outcome (dyspepsia) on top can be drawn to make calculations easier.

	Dyspepsia		
	Yes (n)	No (n)	Total
Drug	6 (A)	38 (B)	44 (A + B)
Placebo	2 (C)	37 (D)	39 (C + D)
Total	8 (A + C)	75 (B + D)	83

This question looks at the chances of developing dyspepsia with sertraline. It is otherwise called the 'experimental event rate' (EER). This is calculated as A/(A + B); that is, 6/44 = 0.136 or 13.6%. Similar to the above question, the chances of developing dyspepsia with placebo, or the 'control event rate' (CER) is C/(C + D), or 2/39 = 0.05 or 5%.

Andrade C. Understanding risk. *Synergy Times* 2001; **1**: 74.

Streiner DL. Risky business: making sense of estimates of risk. Research Methods in Psychiatry. *Canadian Journal of Psychiatry* 1998; **43**: 411–415.

84. C.   This is otherwise called the 'attributable risk' or the 'risk difference' or 'absolute risk reduction' (ARR). It is calculated as the difference in the absolute risks of developing a headache between sertraline and placebo, that is $13.6 - 5 = 8.6\%$

Streiner DL. Risky business: making sense of estimates of risk. Research methods in psychiatry. *Canadian Journal of Psychiatry* 1998; **43**: 411–415.

85. B.   This question asks for the 'relative risk' or 'risk ratio' of dyspepsia with sertraline. It is an estimate of how much greater is the risk of developing dyspepsia with sertraline than with placebo. It is the ratio of the absolute risks or ratio of event rates, i.e. EER/CER = $13.6/5 = 2.7$. This means that the risk of dyspepsia with sertraline is 2.7 times that of placebo. If there is no difference between sertraline and placebo, the relative risk would be 1. Expressed otherwise, relative risk values that are more than 1.0 represent increases in risk. Relative risk values that are less than 1.0 represent decreases in risk. If 95% confidence intervals are given, and if the range includes the value 1, then the elevation in risk can be considered as statistically insignificant. The relative risk is used as a primary summary measure in RCTs and cohort studies.

Streiner DL. Risky business: making sense of estimates of risk. Research methods in psychiatry. *Canadian Journal of Psychiatry* 1998; **43**: 411–415.

86. B.   This question looks at the odds ratio. It is an estimate of how many times more likely it was that a person who experienced a problem (dyspepsia) was exposed to the supposed cause (risk factor) than was a control subject (those not exposed to the risk factor). Let us consider the data in the table in a different way: the number of people who developed dyspepsia is 8 and those who did not develop dyspepsia is 75. The 'odds' of an event happening is the ratio of the probability of its occurrence to the probability of its non-occurrence. So in patients with dyspepsia, the probability of being on sertraline is A/A + C = 6/8 = 0.75. The probability of being on a placebo is C/A + C = 2/8 = 0.25. Therefore the odds of a person with nausea being on sertraline is 0.75/0.25 = 3 or simply A/C. Similarly, we can also calculate the odds of the person 'without dyspepsia' being on sertraline. It is 38/37 (B/D) = 1.02, i.e. the odds of having used sertraline in those who did not have nausea is 1.02. The ratio of these odds is simply called the odds ratio. The ratio = (A/C)/(B/D) or (AD/BC). That is, 3/1.02 or $6 \times 37/2 \times 38 = 222/76 = 2.92$. The odds ratio is interpreted in a manner more or less similar to the relative risk. Confidence intervals are provided and interpreted in the same manner. Odds ratios are usually used in case control studies and in meta-analyses as primary summary measures.

Streiner DL. Risky business: making sense of estimates of risk. Research methods in psychiatry. *Canadian Journal of Psychiatry* 1998; **43**: 411–415.

87. A. As cost-effectiveness analysis has been applied to healthcare, researchers have used predominantly two methods of calculating the summary measure – the average ACER and incremental cost-effectiveness ratio (ICER). The ACER captures the average cost per effect, i.e. cost of treatment/effect of treatment. In this case, the cost of the new psychotherapy is £10,000 and the effect is 50 depression-free weeks. In the above question, the ACER for the new treatment (psychotherapy) will be C/E = 10,000/50 = £200. The ACER for antidepressants from the question will be 5000/45 = £111.

Hoch JS and Dewa CS. A clinician's guide to correct cost-effectiveness analysis: think incremental not average. *Canadian Journal of Psychiatry* 2008; **53**: 267–274.

Hoch JS and Dewa CS. An introduction to economic evaluation: what's in a name? *Canadian Journal of Psychiatry* 2005; **50**: 159–166.

88. A. In contrast to ACER, the ICER reports the ratio of the change in cost to the change in effect (for example $\Delta C/\Delta E$). In plain and simple language, this pretty much translates to the extra cost per extra effect, i.e. $\Delta C/\Delta E$. From the question, we can see $\Delta C = 10,000 - 5000 = 5000$; $\Delta E = 50 - 45 = 5$ weeks. So, $\Delta C/\Delta E = 5000/5 = £1000$. Again in plain language, this would mean that compared with antidepressants, the new treatment would cost an average of 1000 additional pounds per one added depression-free week. In many economic evaluations, the ICER indicates that a new treatment is relatively more costly ($\Delta C > 0$) and relatively more effective ($\Delta E > 0$) than usual care, as in the situation in the question. Now, it is for the decision makers to decide if this additional money is worth spending.

Hoch JS and Dewa CS. A clinician's guide to correct cost–effectiveness analysis: think incremental not average. *Canadian Journal of Psychiatry* 2008; **53**: 267–274.

Hoch JS, and Dewa CS. An introduction to economic evaluation: what's in a name? *Canadian Journal of Psychiatry* 2005; **50**: 159–166.

89. C. An INB calculation determines whether the net benefit of a new treatment outdoes that of usual care. In our case, the net benefit of psychotherapy surpasses the benefit of using antidepressants. In general, the INB is calculated by valuing ΔE in pounds and then subtracting the associated ΔC. This is where the society's willingness to pay for the additional depression week comes into play. INB is calculated using the formula $(\Delta E \times \lambda) - \Delta C$, where λ is society's willingness to pay for a 1-unit gain of effect. In our question, $\Delta E = 5$ weeks; the service managers are willing to pay around £1500/each depression free week (λ – willingness to pay) and ΔC is £5000. So, INB = $(5 \times 1500) - 5000 = 7500 - 5000 = £2500$. The INB equation computes the net value of patient outcome gained in pounds. When the INB is positive, the value of a new treatment's extra benefits ($\Delta E \times \lambda$) outweighs its extra costs (ΔC). In short, society values the extra effect more than the extra cost (i.e. $\Delta E \times \lambda > \Delta C$). Conversely, when the INB is less than 0, society (or your health service management) does not consider the extra benefit worth the extra cost.

Hoch JS and Dewa CS. A clinician's guide to correct cost–effectiveness analysis: think incremental not average. *Canadian Journal of Psychiatry* 2008; **53**: 267–74.

Hoch JS and Dewa CS. An introduction to economic evaluation: what's in a name? *Canadian Journal of Psychiatry* 2005; **50**: 159–166.

90. C.   Resources are scarce and are relative to needs. The use of resources in one way prevents their use in other ways. For example, if a city council decides to build a hospital on a piece of huge vacant land in the middle of the city, the city forgoes the opportunity to benefit from the next best alternative such as selling the land to decrease the current debt or building a shopping mall that would generate additional income for the council. Opportunity cost is assessed in not just monetary or material terms, but in terms of anything which is of value. The opportunity cost of investing in a healthcare intervention is best measured by the health benefits that could have been achieved had the money been spent on the next best alternative intervention. In this example the cost of not providing the 'next best alternative', antidepressant therapy, is the opportunity cost of providing psychotherapy as the first choice treatment.

Palmer S and Rafferty J. Economic notes: opportunity cost. *British Medical Journal* 1999; **318**: 1551–1552.

91. A.   How does a decision maker decide on the willingness to pay (λ)?

The net benefit approach forces decision makers to directly consider the issue of valuing additional patient outcomes. The INB can be computed with various λ s and analysed using multiple regression techniques. How sensitive the results are to the assumed λ value can be gauged using a cost effectiveness acceptability curve (CEAC). The CEAC shows the probability that a new treatment is cost-effective for different values for λ. So in the given question, if λ is £150, the probability of it being cost-effective is >90%. But if the λ is £10, the probability is less than 25%. At the same time, the probability of cost-effectiveness is also >90% if λ was £100. So, it would be sensible for the decision maker to pay £100 for every depression-free day, rather than a £150.

Hoch JS and Dewa CS. A clinician's guide to correct cost-effectiveness analysis: think incremental not average. *Canadian Journal of Psychiatry* 2008; **53**: 267–74.
Hoch JS and Dewa CS. An introduction to economic evaluation: what's in a name? *Canadian Journal of Psychiatry* 2005; **50**: 159–166.

92. C.   This is a receiver operator curve (ROC). Scores on scales are usually considered to be continuous variables. Although dichotomizing continuous data leads to loss of information, in clinical practice, it makes sense to deal with dichotomous variables. For instance, with the new scale in the question, it would make sense if we can differentiate a depressed patient from a non-depressed patient, rather than just saying patient A had a greater score than patient B. In this situation, we should know where the ideal cut-off for the scale is. However, because the distributions of the scores in these two groups most often overlap, any cut-off point that is chosen will result in two types of errors: false negatives (that is, depressed cases judged to be normal) and false positives (that is, normal cases judged to be depressed). Changing the cut-off point will change the numbers of wrong judgements but will not eliminate the problem. The cut-off point also depends on if we want the test to be more sensitive (as in a screening test) or more specific (as in diagnostic tests). The ROC helps us to determine the ability of a test to discriminate between groups and to choose the optimal cut-off point.

Streiner DL and Cairney J. What's under the ROC? An introduction to receiver operating characteristics curves. *Canadian Journal of Psychiatry* 2007; **52**: 121–128.

93.A. The test in question is a 12-item scale that has a potential score ranging from 1 to 12. The sensitivity and specificity of each cut-off score (in this case, there will be 11 possible cut-off scores, as shown in the figure) is calculated with reference to the gold standard used to diagnose depression (in this case, DSM-IV). These pairs of values are plotted, with (1 − specificity) on the x-axis and the sensitivity on the y-axis, yielding the curve in the figure in question. Note that the true positive rate is synonymous with the term sensitivity, the true negative rate is the same as specificity, and the false positive rate means the same as (1 − specificity); they're simply alternative terms for the same parameters. For simplicity, the graph can be depicted as below

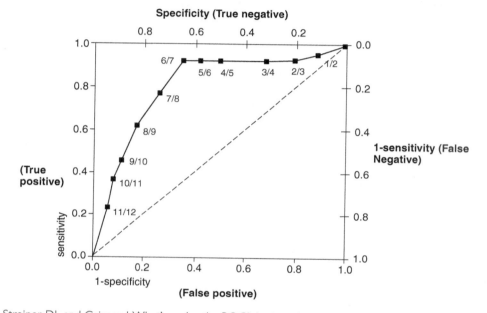

Streiner DL and Cairney J. What's under the ROC? An introduction to receiver operating characteristics curves. *Canadian Journal of Psychiatry* 2007; **52**: 121–8.

94. C. The dotted line represents a test that is useless in discriminating a depressed from a non-depressed person. A perfect test would run straight up the y-axis until the top and then run horizontally to the right. The more the ROC deviates from the dotted line and tends towards the upper left-hand corner, the better the sensitivity and specificity of the test.

Streiner DL and Cairney J. What's under the ROC? An introduction to receiver operating characteristics curves. *Canadian Journal of Psychiatry* 2007; **52**: 121–128.

95. E. From the graph, we can see that the more the ROC curve deviates from the dotted line and tends toward the upper left-hand corner, the better the sensitivity and specificity of the test. Hence it is generally considered that the cut-off point that's closest to this corner is the one that minimizes the overall number of errors ('the best trade off'); in this case, it is 6/7. Since the scale in our question is a screening test for depression, we would want it to be more sensitive rather than specific. As we can see from the figure, a cut-off score of 11/12 would give excellent specificity, but very poor sensitivity, thus increasing the false negative rates.

Streiner DL and Cairney J. What's under the ROC? An introduction to receiver operating characteristics curves. *Canadian Journal of Psychiatry* 2007; **52**: 121–128.

96. C. The primary statistical measure obtained from the ROC is the AUC. The AUC value can be used to compare with the AUC value of a curve corresponding to the null hypothesis. The null hypothesis is represented by a curve that could be obtained if the test has no usefulness in discriminating those with the diagnosis and those without. This hypothetical curve will then have an AUC of 0.50, which corresponds to the area in the graph that falls below the dotted line. The difference in the two AUC consists of the area of the graph between the dotted line and the curve. The AUC can be interpreted in another very useful way. AUC is the probability that the test will show a higher value for a randomly chosen individual with depression than for a randomly chosen individual without depression. That means, if we find the AUC for this particular test was 0.9 and take two individuals at random, one with and one without depression, the probability that the first individual will have a higher score than the second is nearly 90%. Fortunately, the AUC, the sensitivities and specificities, and the whole ROC are calculated by statistical software, sparing us of the burden.

Streiner DL and Cairney J. What's under the ROC? An introduction to receiver operating characteristics curves. *Canadian Journal of Psychiatry* 2007; **52**: 121–128.

97. E.   Meta-analyses are usually displayed in graphical form using Forest plots, which present the findings for all studies plus (usually) the combined results. This allows the reader to visualize how much uncertainty there is around the results. The graph in question, modified below, presents a Forest plot, sometimes called a 'blobbogram' identifying its basic components.

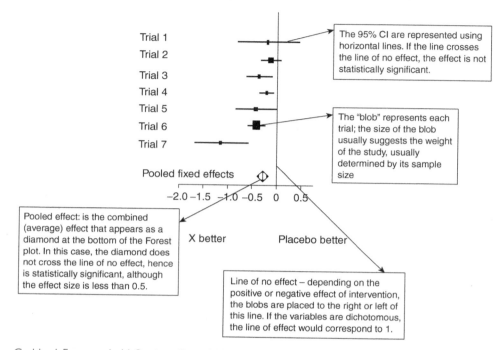

Geddes J, Freemantle N, Streiner D, et al. Understanding and interpreting systematic reviews and meta–analyses. Part 1: rationale, search strategy, and describing results (editorial). *Evidence-Based Mental Health* 1998; **1**: 68–69.

98. C.   As shown in the diagram above, the horizontal lines along with the 'blobs' show the 95% confidence intervals of the effect size or each study. If the confidence intervals cross the line of no effect (at 0 in this case), it suggests that the effect is not statistically significant. Out of the seven studies, the confidence intervals of three of the effect sizes of three of the trials (1, 2 and 5) cross the line of no effect, and four (trials 3, 4, 6 and 7) do not cross the line. The summary measures in cases of dichotomous variables are usually odds ratios, and the line of no effect in that case will correspond to 1.

Perera R and Heneghan C. Interpreting meta–analysis in systematic reviews. *Evidence-Based Medicine* 2008;**13**: 67–69.

99. D.   The size of the blobs (lozenges) in the blobbogram usually represents the size of the study, or more exactly the proportion of the weight that the study contributes to the combined effect. In this case, the largest blob is that of trial 6.

Geddes J, Freemantle N, Streiner D, et al. Understanding and interpreting systematic reviews and meta–analyses. Part 1: rationale, search strategy, and describing results (editorial). *Evidence-Based Mental Health* 1998; **1**: 68–69.

100. D.   A systematic exploration of the uncertainty in the data is known as sensitivity analysis. It is carried out to measure the effects of varying study variables such as individual sample size, number of positive trials, number of negative trials, etc., on expected summary outcome measure of a study (often a meta-analysis or economic study). Sensitivity analysis can be undertaken to answer the question, 'Is the conclusion generated by a meta-analysis affected by the uncertainties in the methods used?' One such uncertainty is publication bias. So, we can use sensitivity analyses to find out the impact of having missed unpublished studies.

Egger M, Davey Smith G, and Phillips A. Meta–analysis: principles and procedures. *British Medical Journal* 1997; **315**: 1533–1537.

Key: ▨ denotes question, ▪ denotes answer